# THE
# BRAZILIAN
# HEALER
## WITH THE
# KITCHEN
# KNIFE

# THE
# BRAZILIAN
# HEALER
## WITH THE
# KITCHEN
# KNIFE

## AND OTHER STORIES OF MYSTICS, SHAMANS, AND MIRACLE-MAKERS

# SANDY JOHNSON

RODALE

© 2003 by Sandy Johnson

Photographs © by James Strachan/Stone/Getty (cover), 2002 Kea Productions (Auntie Margaret), Patty LeGary (Gerry Bostock), Jennifer Emmer (Peter Maxwel)

Printed in the United States of America

Rodale Inc. makes every effort to use acid-free ∞, recycled paper ♻.

Book design by Tara Long

Interior photographs courtesy of Sandra Ingerman, Katie Englehart, Howard Wills, David Reading (Vianna Stibal), Virginia Ellen, Gary Brownlee, Ruth Ziemba, Maki (Rubens Faria), Bob Dinga and Diana Rose (John of God and Ultan).

**Library of Congress Cataloging-in-Publication Data**

Johnson, Sandy.
    The Brazilian healer with the kitchen knife : and other stories of mystics, shamans, and miracle-makers / Sandy Johnson.
        p.    cm.
    ISBN 1–57954–686–2 hardcover
    1. Healers—Popular works.   2. Shamans—Popular works.   3. Mystics—Popular works.   I. Title.
    RZ407.J64   2003
    615.8'52'0922—dc21            2003005804

**Distributed to the book trade by St. Martin's Press**

2  4  6  8  10  9  7  5  3  1  hardcover

Visit us on the Web at www.rodalestore.com, or call us toll-free at (800) 848-4735. For more information about these healers and other books by Sandy Johnson, please visit www.MysticsAndHealers.com.

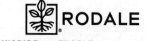

**RODALE**

WE **INSPIRE** AND **ENABLE** PEOPLE TO IMPROVE
THEIR LIVES AND THE WORLD AROUND THEM

*For William M. Johnson, who healed*

# ACKNOWLEDGMENTS

A part from those who allowed me to experience their work and whose stories appear on these pages, I owe a double thanks to Howard Wills. From the beginning, his advice and guidance was invaluable as I navigated these sometimes strange and uncharted seas.

I owe a huge debt of gratitude to Henry Belk and the foundation he left behind. Dr. Bert Schwarz was a constant source of information and encouragement, and Harvey Martin whose book *The Secret Teachings of the Espiritistas* provided vital insight on the Philippine healers.

I am grateful to Bob Dinga and Diana Rose for their photographs of John of God, and to David Sonnenschein who allowed me to quote from his excellent documentary, *Dr. Fritz: Healing the Body and Spirit.*

VIII

My thanks to David Wood, Bob Houston, Joe Naab, and Mark Proteus, who generously shared their experiences with Warren, and to Marty Barigian for providing a photograph of him.

I am grateful to Bill Gray for encouragement and suggestions, Susan Stafford, Cliff Carle for editing assistance, Alex Street for repeated readings and fine-tuning, Sue Terry for research, Shivaya, Dechen Fitzhugh, Juliette Hanauer, David Reading for Vianna's photograph, Maki for his of Rubens Faria, and to Patti LeGary for Gerry Bostock's.

In Brazil, my thanks to Martin Mosquera for his translating skills as well as for his guidance.

My thanks to my agent Bill Gladstone, and to my fine editor, Troy Juliar.

In Hawaii, I am grateful to Nerita Machado, Barbara Moore, Dr. Mimi George, Dr. Mark Lamore, and Ingrid Nelson.

In Los Angeles, my thanks go to the folks at Beyond Physical Therapy, Diane Kehar, Ninfa Bramble, and to Gary Brownlee for their support, physical and non-physical.

And as always, to sons Mark for patient and loving technical support, and Bill and Anthony for never losing faith.

# CONTENTS

# INTRODUCTION

M y travels into the world of mystics and healers began in 1991, when I ceased being an author, mother, teacher, divorcee, hiker, skier, pilot, dog lover—and became a statistic: the one woman in eight diagnosed with breast cancer each year over her lifetime, according to the *Journal of American Medicine*.

I chose the conventional medical route not out of conviction, but out of fear. I knew there were less invasive, less draconian alternatives, and I gave them a hard look. But to choose those roads took courage and unshakable faith, and at the time I did not possess enough of either.

And so, in crisis mode, every nerve in my body on high alert, I entered the world of white-coated wizards with their triple threat treatment: surgery (I opted for a lumpectomy), chemo, and radiation.

In crisis mode there is no place for tears. But then two weeks into chemotherapy on one rare summer day when the mountains were streaked with fiery copper, the sky a shimmering turquoise, I decided to drive out into the desert. With not another car in sight, I could speed along, windows open, and feel the sweet juniper-scented air on my face.

Suddenly I had the strangest sensation. I could feel a whole clump of my hair being ripped from my head. I looked at my side-view mirror and saw it drifting down the road like tumbleweed, stopping when it clung to a cedar tree. I felt another piece of hair fly off. I screeched to a halt at the side of the road, rolled up all the windows, leaned against the steering wheel, and sobbed.

A year-and-a-half later, rounds of treatment completed, the doctor pronounced me cancer-free. Chances of a recurrence would begin to decrease after five years, the doctor explained, and reeled off a timetable of percentages, which I could not hear. Recurrence? Five years? Percentages? I don't call that cancer-free; I call that cancer maybe-if-it doesn't-come-back free.

Fatigued and weak, my head covered with the soft, downy fuzz of a baby chick, my face naked without eyebrows, I felt like a survivor of a bombed-out city, stumbling around in the rubble of my body.

I knew I needed to get strong, and to improve my immune

system so that five or seven years down the road it wouldn't strike again. New Agers, with their theories of why it had happened and what lessons cancer had to teach me made me break out in hives. Yet at the same time I think I knew that as long as there were still demons lurking in the dark corners of my soul real healing might not be possible. Mind, body, and spirit are one. The white-coated wizards had done what they knew how to do to treat—or even cure the disease. But the soul healing would have to come from me.

My sons who had been flying back and forth to be by my side had gone back to their lives; I had a book to finish, one which entailed crisscrossing the country to interview and record the wisdom of the American Indian—much of it by car on unpaved and unmarked reservation roads.

Death had nodded in my direction; I nodded back and moved on. At dawn one morning I got up, packed my tape recorder and notebook, tied a scarf around my awful wig, and took off.

Medicine men and women in various tribes I visited, when they learned I had just been through a life-threatening illness, offered me their own medicines to counteract the effects of chemo and radiation: healing herbs, root extracts used for hundreds of years. And ceremonies. Sweat Lodges in the Plains, all-night Medicine Sings with the Hopi. In the Northeast, I learned to draw a Medicine Wheel. In Colorado, I took peyote that turned my insides out.

Over the next year my hair grew back (a different color), XIII strength returned: perhaps due to the Native medicines, or maybe modern Western science had done its job. In any case, the white-coated wizards were impressed with my lab results. You're fine, they said, go forth and multiply (books, that is).

Soon after the publication of my book on Native American elders, my publisher asked me to write a similar book about Tibetans. Since the Chinese communist invasion in 1950 and subsequent occupation, Tibetans have been living in exile, mostly in India. Dharamsala, in the north, is the seat of the government-in-exile and the current home of the Dalai Lama. I had written His Holiness earlier to request a meeting to discuss my project and gave the dates I expected to be in India. Before the appointed day of my interview, I spent a month getting acquainted with the people of Shangri-La, or in Tibetan, Shambala, the Hidden Kingdom, whose teachings had remained secret for thousands of years.

The similarities between Native Americans and Tibetans were striking. Tibetan oracle-priests and Native American shamans both practice dream-travel, similar ceremonies, meditation, and telepathy. Both cultures also believe in karma, religion as a way of life, and believe that time is circular, non-linear.

My first encounter with mystical healing was with a seventy-five year-old Tibetan nun who had recently escaped the Chinese when they attacked her abbey in Tibet. She lived in a tiny dwelling down the hill from the Dalai Lama's residence. I met her the day before my scheduled appointment with His Holiness, and remember remarking on her apparent good health after such an ordeal. Shaved head, and not a tooth in her mouth, there was something beautiful about her, a radiance, a gleefulness.

Through the translator, she said, "Only a week ago I was blind and couldn't walk." Then she told her story: "We crossed the mountain on foot through snow and ice under cover of dark, just like His Holiness had in 1959. It wasn't until we crossed the border into India that we were taken in and fed and given horses. My whole family had been killed by the Chinese, and many nuns at the abbey had been arrested and tortured, but I had to get to Dharamsala to see the Dalai Lama before I died. For my family. For the other nuns. It was my one wish.

"But when I got here, I was too sick. I couldn't walk, my eyes had gone blind from the snow. And so I just sat here in this little room and meditated. Months went by—I don't know how long—people brought me tea and tsampa [dried barley]—then one day a week ago, two men appeared at my door. They said they had come to take me to see His Holiness. They picked me up and carried me to a car and drove me up the hill to the residence.

"His Holiness welcomed me and called me Ani Gomchen, which means Great Meditator. He stroked my head and recited mantras, and then blew three times on the top of my head.

"All of a sudden I could see! I could look right into his face. And I got up—I stood straight up and walked!" Smiling, her eyes brimming with tears of joy, she stood and took a few long strides to demonstrate. "I walked all the way down the hill to my house."

XV

I remember thinking at the time that the nun's spontaneous healing had been triggered by a state of ecstasy, not unlike the people who throw away their crutches after being tapped on the head by a TV evangelist.

But then the next day, I met with the Dalai Lama. As I sat talking to him and felt the full force of his joy, compassion, and all-encompassing love, I wasn't so sure. And when I got back to my hotel, I noticed the "Delhi-belly" that had felled me the night before, that had me doubled over even into the morning wondering how I would keep my appointment with the Dalai Lama, had completely disappeared. Had my excitement and anticipation of the meeting created an ecstatic state similar to that of the nun's? Or was it in fact the Dalai Lama's famous loving-kindness and compassion that caused my healing?

It seemed my nodding acquaintance with cancer and mortality had set me on a path that would take me through a strange and mysterious maze of smoke and mirrors and bottles of snake oil, and at times send me tumbling down the rabbit hole.

Medical miracles or imagined healings born of an intense desire to believe? Hard to say, but I packed up my laptop, my tape recorder, and my notebook and once again took to the road, this time the road leading to mystics and healers from around the world, determined to solve the mystery.

I've witnessed psychic surgery in Brazil to remove a cancerous tumor without anesthesia from a man's stomach, sleight-of-hand surgery in the Philippines during which the "healer" palmed a piece of chicken liver purchased at the corner stall, and a simple housewife in Florida who goes into a trance and manifests flakes of gold on her skin and, with a second-grade education, quotes medieval French verses. I've also met a housewife-turned-healer in Idaho who commands healings from God.

During my exploration I would experience my own mysterious disappearance of the flu during a healing done over the phone. I would be taken on a shamanic journey to a forest in the "lower world" and to a cloud in the "upper world" and to an event buried deep in my past to meet one of my demons.

And hands so skillful, so intuitive they can only have come directly from the gods. I don't mean laying-on of hands, either, I mean finding the exact location in the body where fear lives. Or grief. Or anger, or loss. The place where toxic tears are stored: fertile ground for illness to take root. And then throwing open the windows of all those dark places and flooding them with air and sunlight.

Celebrity healers who had turned their gift into a multimedia business were of little interest to me, due perhaps to my exposure to the teachings of Native American shamans. They believe that to profit from the gift given by the Great Spirit is to have it taken away or worse, suffer personal punishment. Small donations as tokens of gratitude seemed reasonable, but one healer I came across had people sign a contract promising to pay tens of thousands of dollars in advance.

I also ran across the charlatans (look for the diamond-

encrusted Rolex and the Rolls and the misty-eyed groupies
often called "students"); and the deluded ones, those who truly
believe they are healers, and who with their good intentions and
loving natures often do bring about some sort of a healing—generally not lasting.

But then, seemingly out of nowhere and when least expected,
there is the rare gem: the humble and unfailingly honest miracle-
maker.

# THE BRAZILIAN HEALER WITH THE KITCHEN KNIFE

# CHAPTER
## ONE

# A VISIT

## TO THE LAND

## OF LOST SOULS

### SANDRA INGERMAN

I am just back from India. I go in for my six-month check-up, and my doctor talks to me about support groups. "I already joined the club, I don't need to attend the meetings," I say. "Yes you do," he says. "Do it for them. You're working and living your life. Go let them see. Consider it paying your dues."

Women were already seated in the anteroom of a psychologist's office often used for meditation classes, either on cushions in lotus position or in chairs. Fifteen women in all, in various stages of disease, some in the throes of a recurrence, randomly chosen by fate or karma or a lousy throw of the dice, with little else in common but a desire to say to each other, "I know, I care, here's how I did it."

They look for reasons: "Why me?" they ask, and "What is it

that is keeping me from healing?" They tell stories: of an abusive or neglectful husband, a faithless lover, friends who drew away out of fear or because they just didn't know how to act around them. They feel different, cut off from everyone else in the world who is healthy. They feel alone.

Someone argues that these issues are neither the cause nor the reason for the illness; cancer is not a metaphor for anything, any more than a case of measles or a broken ankle is. It is just cancer. We must find ways to live our lives without waiting for the other shoe to drop.

"No," the facilitator says. "What we have to do is find the hidden source of our illness, that part of our souls that needs healing so that we can be whole again, in mind, body, and spirit."

I think about the many parts of me that are unhealed: the life-long battle with my mother that managed to taint every relationship I ever had, my inability to take charge of my finances. And the many unhealed losses: a brother who died in his 40s of cancer, my father of a sudden heart attack, the good marriage I left for a bad one, and then, just for good measure, one more.

The memory of my best friend who died after a recurrence of breast cancer haunts me. Thirteen years later, at the peak of her career as an actress and married to the love of her life, it snuck up on her like some cruel, cunning thief who stumbled into the wrong house in the middle of the night. She woke up with a cough the next morning. Just a cough.

A woman who had been sitting quietly all evening speaks. "I am an artist, my whole life is my art. But since my operation I'd been unable to pick up a paintbrush. I would lie in bed day after day watching old movies." Until she met a shaman who took her on a spirit journey to find the missing part of her soul and brought it home. "I'm having a show next month," she said. "I hope you'll come."

I asked her which tribe the shaman came from.

She laughed. "The Brooklyn tribe. She's an Anglo from New York living here in Santa Fe. Her name's Sandra Ingerman."

The next day, I passed a bookstore and saw a book in the window, *Soul Retrieval* by Sandra Ingerman, and went in and bought it. A few days later, I was at the gym. The woman on the treadmill next to me looked vaguely familiar. Then I heard a voice call, "Hi, Sandy." I turned, the woman next to me turned. We were both Sandy. The reason she looked familiar was because I had seen her picture on the back of her book, which I had just finished reading. I introduced myself. I told her I had just read her book, she told me she read mine on Native American elders.

Two Sandys, two authors. We made an appointment for the following week.

Sandra lives in a lovely wooded area on the edge of Santa Fe that looks more like the Northeast than the Southwest. A slender woman in her forties, with large dark eyes and long hair, she speaks simply, with traces of New York in her voice.

We sit in the large living room with its expanse of windows that look out onto the dense woods. The trees are filled with birds this time of year, and wildflowers are just beginning to bloom. She talks about her early years, how it was to grow up a child of Depression-era, second-generation Russian parents who were neither religious nor spiritual. The brand of Judaism in her home was more cultural than religious. As a teenager in the sixties, she experimented with LSD and marijuana to try to feed her hunger for some spiritual connection.

"I dropped out of Brooklyn College and migrated to San Francisco. That was in 1972, Haight Ashbury was over, but I didn't know it. I got a job as a bookkeeper for a construction company but soon found out that was not how I wanted to live my life. I got into San Francisco State College in Berkeley and continued on to the California Institute of Integral Studies for a Masters in counseling psychology. I had to hold down two jobs to pay the tuition, working sixty hours a week and running ragged.

"One day somebody came into the registrar's office and said some man from Connecticut was coming to give a weekend workshop. I had no idea who he was or what he was teaching, only that I'd get an extra two credits if I signed up for the workshop. The man turned out to Michael Harner, teaching from his book, *The Way of the Shaman*."

That weekend Ingerman learned how to journey into the spirit world. The experience changed her life.

"On one of those journeys I met my power animal. So many of the questions that had been troubling me for so long were answered. Guilt was my main issue; I had been carrying it around for so long. After that workshop I continued to journey on my own a few times a week. Each time I learned more. Eventually, I could contact my own spirit helpers."

In Native American traditions, a power animal is said to bring "medicine" to whoever calls upon it. Medicine, in this context, is anything—an herb, a crystal, feather, or an animal, that serves to strengthen one's connection to the Great Spirit and to assist in healing. Each animal brings its own kind of medicine: A coyote is said to remind us not to take ourselves too seriously; what seems to be folly may turn out to be wisdom. A horse represents the freedom and power of movement, while the butterfly is the dance of joy. The snake is an archetype of the cycles of death and rebirth. Power animals also act as escorts to the spirit world.

"There are many levels in the spirit world," Sandra explains. "The Lower World, Upper World, and the Middle World. The Lower World is reached through a tunnel that leads into the earth. That landscape is filled with mountains, deserts, seas, and dense jungles. The Upper World is ethereal. The light there tends to be bright, and the colors go from soft pastels to complete darkness. In the Upper World, I know I'm standing on

7

something but I can't feel the earth below my feet. I might find myself walking through a crystal city or floating through the clouds.

"The Middle World is the spiritual side of our ordinary world, and is used by shamans to find lost or stolen objects and to perform long-distance healings."

When it came time for Ingerman to begin her private counseling practice, she found that by incorporating spiritual journeying into her practice, clients became empowered to find their own answers. "Soul retrieval and psychotherapy work incredibly well together. One of the reasons therapy is not always effective is because the therapist is talking to someone who's not really there. Soul retrieval brings the person home, so the psychotherapeutic process can really begin."

Within a few years, Michael Harner invited Ingerman to join the faculty of his foundation. She began to teach and give workshops, gaining a following of her own. A shaman, it seems, can grow just as easily in Brooklyn as in the Plains of South Dakota.

"The word 'shaman' is an ancient word, its roots in Siberia in the Tungus language. It means a healer who sees in the dark. Shamanic journeys have been practiced in cultures all over the world for thousands of years. According to shamanic beliefs, one of the major causes of illness is soul loss, which can occur at the time of severe accident, emotional trauma, even surgery. A part of the soul flees the body to escape the pain or shock.

"This is not necessarily a bad thing. It's a way for the body and psyche to survive severe trauma. The last place the soul wants to be at the time of an accident is in the body. But problems develop when the part of the soul that left doesn't come back. It may have gone out so far and so fast that it can't find its way back. For instance, if a part of the soul left because of child abuse, it might not want to come back.

"In today's society, soul loss usually manifests as a symptom psychologists call dissociation—when people feel that they're watching life as if it's a movie and they're the observer. In clinical terms, dissociation is the separation of whole segments of the personality from the mainstream of consciousness, which can result in feelings of estrangement and depersonalization. For example, incest survivors often remember the experience of being raped or abused from the perspective of looking down at their bodies.

"Coma is an extreme example of soul loss; when the entire soul leaves the body, the body dies. People who have had serious accidents frequently recall out-of-body experiences."

Ingerman told of three of her own near-death experiences, which according to Michael Harner marked her entry into shamanism. At seven, she was hit by lightning; at nineteen, she nearly died in a drowning incident off the coast of Mazatlán, Mexico. "I was drowning, I felt myself go into the light, to God. There was a garden, a place so spectacular words can't describe. And again when I was twenty-six, in a car accident. The car went off a cliff on a mountain road. There was no reason why

9

any one of us in that car should be alive, but miraculously no one was hurt.

"In that moment, I learned we live in a loving universe, that when you go to the light, God doesn't know whether you're a good person or a murderer. There is no judgment, there is only love. No heaven, no hell, no sin. The purpose of organized religion, as I saw it, was to get people to behave. God doesn't see us as individuals; we are all one. Life was never the same for me after those experiences.

"When I first started my shamanic healing practice, ten or fifteen years ago, most of my clients were cancer patients. I was the last stop on the train. I saw some incredible reversals, but I've had no success with AIDS."

I asked her if she can tell when someone has had a soul loss.

"A common symptom is when someone tells me they feel spaced out all the time, or can't remember certain traumatic events, or even entire periods of their lives. I can understand not remembering things that happened before the age of five, but when a person can't remember even one day of being nine, that's a signal something is wrong.

"Another symptom of probable soul loss is when people have themes that go on throughout their lives, such as not being able to trust. Addiction, too. I've found that when people have lost soul parts, they might try to fill themselves with something external to avoid feeling the emptiness inside.

"Chronic illness may also be an indication of soul loss. If people are not fully in their bodies, they may not be vital enough to protect themselves from different illnesses. Chronic depression could be another symptom, although that could also be caused by power loss."

I asked about power loss and how it is different from soul loss.

"Core shamanism," Sandra explains, "teaches that we all have power animals around us who protect us and keep us healthy. If a power animal goes away and another one doesn't come in to take its place, we experience a loss of power, which could lead to chronic problems such as depression, illness, or misfortune.

"Shamanism cures, but the person has to do the healing."

She then asks me if I would like to go on a shamanic journey with her.

I hesitate; not because I'm not curious, I am. But in the past when I've been taken on a guided meditation and thought I heard or saw things, I couldn't quite trust whether it was coming from inside my own head or from someplace else. And in the spirit of cooperation I would go along with it, never really trusting the process.

Sandra smiles, stands. "C'mon," she says, "Let's just see what happens."

I follow her through her living room, dining room, and down a hallway to the few steps that descend to a darkened room that is her office.

It is a room filled with her sacred objects: a flute, drums, Kachina dolls, animal fetishes, gourds, feathers, dream-catchers, crystals, candles, incense, drums. Many of the objects I recognize 11 from my own travels. She shows me a carved horn made of bone with a rope attached that is used by Northwest coast people to capture lost souls, and a rattle carved from a gourd. From outside the window, chimes ring softly. Sandra puts on a tape of a flute playing a haunting tribal melody.

On the floor in the center of the room is a burgundy and gray Mexican Zapotec rug. Sandra tells me we will use that to lie on during the journey. She lights a candle. "This is to call on the helping spirits," she says. Then she places a crystal, a drum, and a rattle on the blanket. Even though the drumming comes from a shamanic tape, she likes to have the drum nearby, as another ceremonial symbol.

The journey begins. I am asked to close my eyes and to take some deep, cleansing breaths. Then Sandra kneels next to me and begins to whistle, calling to the spirits, and using the rattle as accompaniment, she sings out. Then, when she has reached her altered state, she lies next to me. I have been instructed to lie quietly and to stay as present and receptive as possible.

The drumbeats on the tape grow louder, faster. They seem to become one with my own heartbeat. After a time, the sound becomes the beat of hooves pounding the earth. In my mind I see a white horse standing before me. He whinnies and paws the earth, and with a shake of his head he beckons to me. I see myself walking toward him. Grabbing onto his thick white mane, I pull myself onto his back.

I feel myself about to question what I am seeing, but no, I force myself to stay with it.

The horse turns and begins to gallop into the night. I feel liberated, released. I laugh out loud. We soar, my white stallion and I, up through the stars, above the night to a space that is all light.

In the distance is a tiny flame. It grows larger as we approach, larger still, until it is a fire. A huge fire. I yank the mane with all my strength but the horse does not stop.

I realize it is a house. The house of my childhood.

Suddenly, I am standing alone in the middle of my room, crying. I am six years old. I have been put in my room by my mother to punish me. I go to the window and watch her car disappear down the driveway.

I smell smoke. I turn and see it curl underneath my door. I call out. No one hears me.

Enough. I don't like this.

I feel Sandra's hand on my arm as I start to get up. "Stay," she whispers. "Stay."

Flames shoot out at me. Then the door smashes open. A man rushes in. Black shiny suit, hat. A fireman. He puts a blanket over my face and carries me down the stairs. Then I am outside in my father's arms. My mother is not there.

Tears trickle along my cheeks into my ears. Sandra is bringing me to a sitting position. Kneeling behind me, she blows on the top of my head. The coolness of her breath brings a tingling sensation to my scalp. She shakes the rattle four times around my body. I tell her about the images I saw. She explains that a part

13

of my soul had fled my body then, escaping to survive the ordeal and leaving my body vulnerable to illness. In her altered state, Sandra had traveled to the spirit world, located it, and brought it back. Now she was blowing that part of my soul back into my body through the crown of my head. Shaking the rattle, she welcomed it home.

When I sit up, I look at her. I do not understand what happened, but I do know I didn't conjure it. Certainly not consciously. Sandra says she saw the horse, and that he is my power animal. She also saw me at five or six, frightened and crying. And that then is when part of my soul took off.

She asks me how I feel. I wish I could say I suddenly feel whole, but Sandra assures me I will feel a shift in the days to come.

I feel dazed. I try to remember the fire. I wonder where my brother was during the fire? If I was six, my brother, four years older, must have been at some sort of after-school sports practice. But we had a nanny-housekeeper, where was she? I have no one to ask. My brother and father have both passed away. I call my cousin who is my age. She remembers only vaguely something about a fire, and my family going to live with our grandparents. An aunt on my father's side thinks she remembers hearing something about a fire, too.

Wait a minute—I was left alone in the house to perish in a fire and nobody remembers? No wonder my soul took a powder.

I decide I will ask my mother next time I visit her in Florida. Immediately though, the thought causes a twinge in my

stomach. Conversations of that sort do not typically go well between us.

I try to visualize the horse again, as Sandra suggested, to let
him be my power animal. Often when I am walking and trying
to solve a problem, I try to imagine him walking beside me. And
when I stop and sit beneath a tree and close my eyes, I imagine
myself climbing onto his back and letting him take me wherever
he thinks we should go.

But we never again go back to that fire.

Do I feel as if I've been made whole again? I can't honestly
say I do. But maybe it's a start.

# CHAPTER
# TWO

# KATIE'S

# GOLD

## KATIE ENGLEHART

I always made my mother angry. My hair could make her angry, or my clothes, the places I chose to live, the books I wrote—she took it all as a personal affront. "You were the only person in my life I couldn't control," she once said. That summed it up, I suppose.

A host of ailments plagued her: macular degeneration, a progressive disease that would one day cause total blindness; painful arthritis in both knees, which she bore with maddening stoicism; and I noticed lately when we spoke on the phone she had difficulty hearing.

On the plane on the way down, I rehearsed the question I would put to her about the fire over and over in my mind, trying to find a way to phrase it in a way that would not be perceived as confrontational.

Bad mother-daughter relationships are a cliché; ours is of biblical proportions. Still, I kept on believing if I tried hard enough—short of total surrender on my part—that I could find a way to unlock her heart. Over the years I had tried many keys, and none of them worked.

Predictably, when I told her about my current interest in mystical healing, she shook her head like the angry Queen. "That's ridiculous," she said. "There's no such thing. If there were, don't you think medical science would know about it?"

I had another reason for my trip to Florida: I had been in touch with Dr. Bertrand Schwarz in Vero Beach, an hour or so north of Palm Beach. Author of over 160 articles for various scientific journals, graduate of Dartmouth and NYU, a four-year Fellow at Mayo Clinic, Dr. Schwarz, who had a thriving psychiatric practice, had been investigating psychic phenomenon and energy healing for more than forty years.

Tall and slender with a courtly manner and silver hair and mustache, he looked like an elegant 19th-century gentleman. His office was furnished like a museum: forty years of books, photographs, videos, audio tapes, and various objects that Dr. Schwarz referred to as "apportations," a term used in psychic writings to describe the phenomenon of solid objects appearing, teleported, through matter. I asked him about the large glass jar filled with what appeared to be gold flakes.

The doctor took it down and showed it to me. "These came

off of the surface of a woman's skin, materialized while she was in a trance," he said.

Katie Englehart, a thirty-seven-year-old housewife and part-time cleaning woman, first came to his office in 1987 after repeated trance-induced events that terrified her and embarrassed her family. Once, while waiting in line at a convenience store, and another time at a restaurant, she had gone into a spontaneous trance and within seconds golden flakes began to appear on her upper lip and forearms.

During their first session, Dr. Schwarz asked Katie if she could go into a trance at will. She said she'd try. The doctor watched as her eyes fluttered. Moments later, flakes of gold appeared on her face, neck, hands, chest and back, flakes large enough that the doctor could peel them off. Afterward, Katie said she had the taste of copper in her mouth.

Schwarz put the flakes in a jar and sent them off for chemical analysis. The chemist's report came back with an analysis of 98 percent copper and 2 percent zinc. The zinc gave the substance its goldlike appearance. The doctor asked Katie if he might record and videotape her trances during subsequent visits.

During one session, Katie, who had no more than a second-grade education, began to write verses in medieval French. Dr. Schwarz had the verses translated by a language scholar who found them to be letter-perfect in grammar and spelling. He showed me a sample of one written in handwriting resembling an eight-year-old's:

19

*Perdu Trouve, cache*
*De si long siecle sera*
*Pasteur demi honore*
*Aina quela la . . . [unfinished]*


*Lost, found, hidden*
*For such long centuries will be*
*The half-honored shepherd*
*Thus, until the . . .*


"I just saw the letters in my mind's eye," Katie explained.

During other visits, Dr. Schwarz realized Katie possessed the ability to see into the future and to heal. According to Dr. Schwarz, a seventy-eight-year-old man, the father of a friend of Katie's and a doctor himself, asked Katie if she thought she might be able to help him with his deafness and arthritic knees. She said she didn't know, but agreed to try.

One day, at his son's home, Katie placed her hands on the father's knees and then on his ears. Twenty minutes later, tiny gold flecks appeared around the man's ears and knees.

The man's wife said Katie must be a witch. They called Dr. Schwarz to tell him what had happened. For the first time in months the man began to walk two miles every day, and his hearing improved dramatically.

Some months later, in the evening, Dr. Schwarz stopped by his office to check his messages. There were three from Katie.

Her voice was frantic. "Doc, this is Katie. It's happening all over again. The pen is absolutely standing up by itself and writing. The whole place is shaking . . . it's writing!" The second message had Katie shouting, "Mine and Mike's pictures are stuck to the wall . . . when the pen started writing . . . the picture . . . whooshed to the wall. It's just hanging there! We're waiting for it to fall . . ."

The third message was from Katie's teenaged son, Mike. "Come back, Doc, other stuff is going on."

When Dr. Schwarz arrived, the Polaroid picture was stuck to the wall; the doctor gently touched it and it fell. No adhesive was on the back or on the wall. Katie was standing in the dining room, twelve feet away, watching the pen write on a piece of paper on the round, glass-topped table in the family room. The house shook; their German shepherd went wild and barked ferociously.

The doctor took the sheet of paper with Katie's large, scrawled writing and had it translated:

> *Plui, faim, guerre en*
> *Perse non cessee,*
> *La foi trop grand*
> *trahira le monargue:*
> *par la Finie en Gaule*
> *commencee,*
> *secret augure pour a un*
> *estre pargue.*

*Rain, hunger, no end to war in Persia,*
*Over-confidence will betray the monarch:*
*it will end in Gaul where it began,*
*secret omen for a fated being.*

"Katie has no desire to convince or impress others," Dr. Schwarz explained. "She doesn't remember much of what happens to her in trance, and she is so busy with her family and job that she apparently seldom thinks of these matters when she is working."

I said I would like very much to meet her.

Dr. Schwarz called Katie to ask if she were free to see me that afternoon.

Katie lived with her husband and teen-aged son in a tract house a few miles from Dr. Schwarz. Simply furnished and neat as a pin, the house reflected Katie's warmth and unpretentiousness. She told me she did not fancy herself "chosen" or having "the gift." She just shrugged and smiled and in her pleasant Tennessee twang said, "I don't know myself how or why these things happen to me, but if it helps anyone I'm glad."

The "things" she referred to had happened to her all her life. Born in the mountain hamlet of Copperhill, Tennessee, daughter of a miner and tenth of twelve children, Katie had to leave school in the second grade to take care of her paralyzed mother.

"I learned to cook and clean and haul water from the time I was eight years old, but I never learned to read and write—except my name. And I know numbers, but I'm not very good at math."

I asked if I might turn on my tape recorder. "Sure," she said, "but I can't promise I'll say anything worth recording."

After fifteen or twenty minutes, just when I thought the whole tape would be used up on pleasant chit-chat, Katie stopped talking and began to rub her left knee. She frowned as if in pain. "Are you all right?" I asked.

Katie winced, and her eyes glazed over.

"Your mother," she said. "You need to rub her knee with some nice oil . . . skin's so dry . . . show her you care. . . . She loves you, but her love is locked away somewhere inside and she can't get to it." Katie paused; her eyes unfocused exactly like my mother's.

I stared at her, speechless, not daring to move.

Suddenly she sprang to her feet. "Would you like something to drink? Iced tea or a Coke? I'm real thirsty."

I looked up at her. "How's your knee?"

"My knee? There's nothing wrong with my knee—why?"

"Katie, do you remember what you just told me about my mother?"

She frowned, shook her head. The last thing she remembered talking about was the lady down the street whose dog was about to have puppies.

I sped back to my mother's. What had I just seen? Why had Katie tuned into my mother so accurately? Had she passed away and was speaking to me through Katie?

23

But there she was, standing in the living room, leaning on her walker, being awful to Jan, her caregiver. "Hello, Mother," I called out.

A curt greeting, then she told me I had a phone call.

"From who?" I asked.

"I don't know. I can't see to take a message."

"Why didn't you let Jan take the call?"

"Go get ready for dinner," she said. "You look terrible."

"Mother, if you can't see to take a telephone message, how do you know I look terrible?"

"Sandy, please don't stand there arguing with me. Go get ready for dinner."

Her love is locked away, I told myself as I went to my room. It is definitely locked away.

That night, when I went to her room to say goodnight, I found her sitting in her chair, the TV tuned to a sitcom.

"What are you watching?"

"I don't know," she said irritably.

I remembered what Katie said. "Would you like me rub your knee?"

Her eyes tried to find me. After a moment, she said, "Yes. I would."

I went and got some lavender oil and sat on her footstool. I began to massage it in. Her knee was swollen, the skin so dry and cold it almost didn't feel like flesh at all, not living flesh.

It repelled me; I wanted to pull away. Then I looked up at her.

Her eyes were closed, her face relaxed. I am of this flesh, I thought. And yes, even of this soul.

My mother opened her eyes, and I could tell for a moment they focused on me. "Your hair looks nice," she said softly.

The next morning, out on the patio where I was having coffee, I turned at the sound of my mother's walker on the marble floor. I noticed she did not seem to be putting all that much weight on the walker so I asked her about it. "Strangest thing," she said. "My knee feels so much better. I think that oil you put on it last night must have helped."

I leaned over to have a closer look, half-expecting to see Katie's gold on her knee.

"I'm glad," I said.

Maybe next time I would ask her about the fire.

# CHAPTER
# THREE

# DISTANCE

# HEALING

## HOWARD WILLS

B ert Schwarz had gone through his files and drawn up a list of people whose work he had studied over the years.

"Here's someone who can do distance healing—over the phone."

Had it been anyone other than the highly creditable, buttoned-down and pinstriped Dr. Schwarz, I surely would have rolled my eyes at the suggestion that someone could possibly effect a healing over the telephone.

"You mean like a TV remote?" I asked. "Or e-mail traveling back and forth across through the ether?"

"Or like the PET scan or MRIs. The principle behind those

devices that at one time would have been considered science fiction had been hiding in plain sight for decades."

Hard to imagine, but until a week ago I'd never heard of gold coming off a person's skin, either. I grabbed for a pencil.

When I called to introduce myself and explained my project, Howard Wills told me he planned to be in the Los Angeles area in a few weeks—which happened to coincide with when I planned to be there. He invited me to attend one of his sessions in Topanga Canyon, at a place where he gives healings. Afterward, we would have a chance to talk.

Howard Wills was born in 1953 in Columbia, South Carolina, the second of six children. His father owned the furniture factory that would one day pass to him. His mother, raised in a Catholic orphanage, was deeply religious and "forever praying."

Howard's boyhood was plagued by illnesses. Pneumonia landed him in a hospital when he was five. He remembers feeling himself looking down from above and seeing his body lying inside an oxygen tent and wondering why he had gotten so sick. "If my body knows how to get sick," he remembers thinking, "it must know how to get well, too."

That thought stayed with him. At twelve he wanted to know about the herbs the American Indians out in the countryside used to treat the sick. And the blacks who seemed to have ways of their own. Howard went to them and asked questions.

By the time he was twenty, a student at the University of

South Carolina, he knew what he wanted to do. He wanted to learn how to help people with their healing, but he did not know how to go about it. Until the day the answer came to him, presumably from a spirit.

He was walking across campus between classes when he thought he heard a voice. He looked around. It was a voice, and it was speaking to him, clear and plain. It told him to go up on that hill and lie down. "Take off your shoes and align yourself with the sun. Turn your palms up and look at the sun, breathe in its light, let the light fill your body, let your body become a cocoon of light."

Some time went by, and Howard lost consciousness. Three hours later he woke up and checked his watch. He had missed two classes. Still groggy, he looked down at the people walking along the sidewalk at the bottom of the hill. He shook his head and looked again. They were transparent. It was as if they were made of cellophane. My God, he thought, I'm seeing right through these people! Their systems looked like an electric grid with intersecting lines, all in different colors.

In a moment their bodies were back to normal. Then, a few days later, they became transparent again, but this time they appeared to Howard as egg-shaped sacs filled with water. Howard never told anyone what he had heard and seen that day on campus, not for twenty more years.

I asked my friend Adam Rodman, a screenwriter who has been plagued with a bad back for years, if he'd like to come with 29 me. Skeptical but curious, he said he would gladly welcome a miraculous healing, even though he had serious doubts it could be done in his case.

Topanga Canyon, nestled in the Santa Monica Mountains high above the beaches of Malibu, is a community frozen in time. Artists, filmmakers, poets, and writers, their hair streaked with gray now instead of flowers—they are the remnants of counter-culture of the sixties, now with children of their own.

We drive along the Pacific Coast Highway, beach on our left, and beyond, the astounding blue of the Pacific dotted with black-suited figures on surfboards skimming the waves. We wind our way up the canyon road, past log cabin stores, a co-op grocery, the rustic Theatricum Botanicum, an outdoor theater founded by the actor Will Geer. We cross a painted bridge and turn off onto a narrow, steep uphill road and look for a sign: Center for Spiritual Studies. Dozens of cars jam three makeshift parking areas. It seems Howard Wills packs them in.

The house was built in the sixties and added onto over the years to accommodate the steady stream of spiritual masters, teachers, and healers invited to hold their programs and ceremonies on the property.

Outside, children swing from a tire hung from a tree, dogs chase each other, a man in a ponytail lies in a hammock reading, a white-robed Indian holding a strand of beads strolls, deep in meditation. Down the hill, construction workers are putting up a yurt. Buzz saws and hammers blend in with sounds of wind chimes, birdsongs, dogs barking, and from inside a tape playing Indian chants.

On the veranda, beneath colorful Tibetan prayer flags, are rows of shoes: Birkenstocks, clogs, rubber sandals. Adam and I lean down to untie our out-of-place sneakers and walk through the kitchen to a large, windowed room.

Twenty-five or thirty people sit in a semicircle around Howard Wills. Beneath the window is an altar covered with an Indian cloth. On it are lighted candles, flowers, incense, a framed photograph of an Indian saint.

Howard, blue-eyed, dark-haired, is dressed in white slacks and white shirt. His smile is boyish, charismatic. He smiles at us as we slip into chairs at the back of the room. "Hi, how y'all doin'?" His drawl is part southern, part good ol' boy.

Next to Howard, a seventeen-year-old boy, paralyzed from a car accident, sits in a wheelchair. His sister has flown in from Hawaii to bring him here.

Howard turns and speaks softly to the boy. "How you feelin' now? You're gonna walk today, aren't you? We're goin' to do it together, right?"

The boy smiles, head tilted to the side, and makes a sound.

We watch silently. This boy could be any of us, or one of our children. Out of nowhere, a crash, sirens, a wheelchair. With all our hearts we want to see a miracle.

Howard stands behind the boy and places his hands on the boy's shoulders, and closes his eyes. Then, he points to the boy's

31

legs and begins to blink rapidly for several minutes. No one moves, barely drawing a breath.

32

Then Howard leans over and looks into the boy's eyes. "Now in a few minutes you and I are goin' to take a little walk, okay?"

The boy gives Howard his lopsided smile and nods his head.

After a moment, Howard takes his seat and looks around the room. He knows some of the people by name. "Hey, Sue, how are those headaches?"

Sue nods. "Much better. I haven't had a migraine for a month now, since the last time you were here."

"Good! How 'bout you, Barbara? You doin' any better today?"

The woman next to her looks up, tears in her eyes, and says quietly, "I think so."

A man sitting on a cushion against the wall has been diagnosed with a small tumor in his lung. He will undergo an operation, but before he does, he wants to see if Howard's healing can shrink the tumor.

Howard comes over to Adam. Adam explains his problem with his back. Howard asks him to stand and bend over as far as he can. He bends halfway. Howard asks if he'd like to fix that, Adam answers, "Oh yes."

"Well good then, let's fix it."

After Howard has made the rounds, speaking to each

person, sometimes placing a hand on a shoulder or a head, he takes his seat and leads the group in a series of eight prayers beginning with an ancestral prayer ". . . to dissolve karma of past and present lives that causes physical and spiritual illness, and to open awareness of mind and heart," ending with a prayer of thanks.

I look around the room at the faces of those repeating the prayers, faces full of hope and of faith. I change my mind: These people are not hippie artifacts; they are not even New-Agers; these are people of the new spirituality who know that nothing in this new world is sure or safe or permanent. Howard is like a magnet, a lightning rod for the deep, primal longing in each of us to connect with whatever power or force we believe in. Whatever name we give to it, we want our lives to be touched by it.

After the prayers, Howard turns back to the boy in the wheelchair.

"What d'you think? You ready to try now?" There is goodness in his smile; the boy feels it and smiles back. Awkwardly, his hand hanging limp, he reaches for Howard.

"All right, then. Here we go." From behind, Howard gets the boy to his feet. His leg braces clank as he struggles to get up. The room is silent. Outside, even the buzz saw has stopped; the wind has stilled the chimes. The only sound is that of the sitar playing a plaintive tune on a tape.

It is almost too painful to watch.

33

Howard holds onto him as they take some halting steps across the room. Then Howard, sensing it is all the boy can do, helps him back into his wheelchair.

I look over at the boy's sister. She has been watching intently. For a brief moment, hope flickered in her eyes; then, when he sat back down she smiled reassuringly and patted his hand.

Howard explains they will repeat this process several times throughout the day, and for each of the four days Howard is there.

But it is clear that on this day we will not witness a miraculous healing.

In my mind the healing has failed. I wonder how Howard views it. After the session, I ask him.

"Sometimes healing happens in minutes, other times it's a longer process. I'm not the healer, it's God who does the healing. I'm just the janitor. I clean out the muck that caused the illness in the first place."

I ask him what is happening when he blinks his eyes and points.

"I'm assisting the person to receive light. Where someone is disconnected, I'm making the connection."

I do not quite understand. I press him for a fuller explanation and, patiently, he repeats the statement. Feeling I am stepping on hallowed ground, I withdraw the question. Howard tells me these are mysteries that cannot be explained, implying that it is foolishness to try.

In the car on the way back, I ask Adam how his back feels. He tells me it feels better, that he has a greater range of motion. He thinks something may have happened. Adam likes Howard; he feels he is sincere and believes he is gifted.

A few days later, when I call Adam to ask about his back, he tells me he felt a definite improvement. A week later though, the pain and stiffness have returned. When I call and speak to Howard about this, he says, "Adam has to remember to do the prayers I gave him." If Howard has a magic bullet, it comes with instructions.

On another day, a man and wife, Bob and Hermina Rasmussen, drive to L.A. from their home in Paso Robles, in Northern California—a four-hour drive. Bob, eighty-one and considered by many a beloved master healer, had gone blind in 1997, a result of diabetes. One of the founders of the early energy healing movement in California, Bob had published two books and, over the years, given seminars to more than 4,000 students throughout the U.S. and Switzerland. Film studios called on him to work on stunt men injured during shooting or actors taken ill. To Bob Rasmussen, the gift of healing was a grace. But as was the case of many healers I had spoken to, he could not heal himself.

Instead he had come to accept his fate in a Zen-like way, but for the past few days he had been telling his wife Hermina, that his dream was to regain his sight—for just one day before he died. Hermina, younger by twenty-one years, would do anything to help him have his dream.

As if on cue, a phone call from a trusted friend came telling them about an incredible healer in South Carolina. Hermina called Howard Wills right away. When she heard he would be in Los Angeles the very next day, they were elated. It was a sign.

The Rasmussens got into their car at nine in the morning and arrived at the center in Topanga at one-thirty. Howard was on a lunch break. They waited, Hermina nervous, Bob full of hope. He repeated his wish. "If I could only see—for just one day . . ."

On that particular day some other healers had come to watch Howard's work. The session proceeded as usual, Howard going around the room, greeting each person, asking how they were doing. When he came to Bob and learned that he was a healer who had lost his sight, he got to work.

Hand extended but not touching him, Howard stood a few feet in front of Bob. To many in the room, the laser-like energy passing from Howard to Bob was palpable. Twenty minutes later, in a moment no one present will forget, Howard held up two fingers. "How many fingers do you see, Bob?"

Bob gasped. "I see two. I see two fingers!"

Howard held up three fingers. "Now how many?"

"Three!"

Hermina wept. People who had witnessed dozens of healings were moved to tears. On this day, Howard had indeed produced a miracle.

That afternoon, Bob and Hermina started for home. On the way they stopped at an outdoor restaurant for a late lunch. Their table overlooked a river; on the other side, the tree-shrouded mountainside rose up, splashed with feathery lipstick-red blossom. Bob devoured it all with his eyes—the yellow and white wildflowers on the table, the color and texture of the food; most of all, he could see the face of his wife.

He fell asleep that night, happiest he had been in four years.

The next morning, he woke up and lay quiet. Then, softly, he said to Hermina, "It's gone. It's all black again."

Eight months later, after a series of strokes, Bob Rasmussen died.

But he had gotten his wish. For just one day, he could see.

In July, I flew to New Mexico for the birth of a grandson, my son and daughter-in-law's first baby. Melanie had been having contractions for two days and Anthony was a wreck. The morning she finally went into labor and Anthony rushed her to the hospital, I woke up with a raging sore throat. I recognized it at once. It was the kind that invariably turns into a head cold, then takes up a month-long residence in the chest.

My bones and muscles ached: I was in for it. I would have to leave without even seeing the baby for fear of contamination. Utterly miserable, I got out my bag and started to pack. Then I

37

thought of Howard. A far-fetched idea, but why not try? I called him at his furniture factory and apologized for bothering him, then explained my dilemma.

"That's okay, darlin'," he drawled, "Give me a minute, hold the phone and look out the window at the sky. Can you see it?"

"I can see it."

"Okay, hold on."

Silence. Three or four minutes went by. This is ridiculous; I'm really losing it.

"Swallow," Howard said.

I swallowed. My throat was on fire. My head hurt, everything hurt.

"How does that feel?" he asked. I was tempted to say "fine," and let the man get back to building mattresses. I didn't, though.

"Sorry," I said. "But thanks anyway."

"Wait a minute, honey. Let's try again."

Another few minutes, then he asked me to swallow again. Nothing. I thanked him and said goodbye. I got out my airline ticket to change my flight. I dialed the number, but as I started to speak I realized my throat had stopped hurting. Not only that, but my head had stopped throbbing. And the aches were gone!

Call it placebo, call it madness, I didn't care. I didn't have to leave. That afternoon, I held my baby grandson.

Later on, when I questioned Howard, he explained that in the world of spirit, time and distance do not exist. His spirit had been able to connect with mine. And with the force of his intention and his ability to send loving energy, I had gotten healed. "Pure physics," he said with a chuckle in his voice.

It was useless to try to make sense of it; reason doesn't work here. One has to make the leap through the looking glass and over the rainbow, beyond the world's horizons, and even then be willing to believe the unbelievable.

Every culture throughout history has created stories to try to explain the mystery of life and death, illness and healing. I am reminded of a quote attributed to John La Farge, son of the American painter, upon visiting the French shrine of Lourdes and observing the cures: "For those who believe in God no explanation is necessary; for those who do not, no explanation is possible."

# CHAPTER
# FOUR

# HEALER,
# HEAL THYSELF

## VIANNA STIBAL

I had been hearing about Vianna Stibal from people involved in the alternative healing world for months. Described as an Idaho housewife who performs distance healings that are said by many to be nothing less than miraculous, I was eager to meet her. It took a few months before I finally got through to her on the phone (she gets two hundred calls a week). When I finally did reach her she greeted me like an old friend. Her voice was warm and intimate and charmingly lighthearted. Like Howard's.

But unlike Howard, Vianna doesn't believe in asking God for help; she commands God. "Asking gets the subconscious deciding whether or not you deserve what you want, but when you use the words 'I command,' your subconscious accepts that because you are a part of God, you have a divine right to choose

what you want. By commanding God, you are stepping into the role of co-creator."

Vianna told me that for her it was a matter of survival. She describes her childhood as "sad." Her parents divorced when she was three. Her mother, a Baptist who converted to the Mormon Church, married several times, moving her children from state to state. At fifteen, Vianna dropped out of school; by sixteen she was married.

The marriage did not last. After her divorce, Vianna went back to school to get her high school diploma, then on to college. Poor and on welfare, she hunted for food, learned to shoot deer.

At twenty-seven, a divorced mother of three, Vianna got a job as a security guard at a local manufacturing plant. During breaks she would sit and draw sketches of the other employees. As she studied their faces she had sudden flashes of intuition about their health and would tell them what she saw. The accuracy of her readings amazed them. Vianna, realizing she had some natural gift she didn't quite understand, decided to study naturopathy and massage to become a full-time health practitioner. Eventually, her intuitive readings became more and more a part of her practice.

Four years later, in the summer of 1995, Vianna's right leg suddenly began to swell, causing her terrible pain. Within weeks the leg had swelled to twice its normal size. After a series of tests, doctors diagnosed her with advanced bone cancer. They said they would have to amputate the leg to prevent the spread of the disease. She might not have more than three or four months to live.

Vianna wasn't sure the doctors were right. She told the doctors the exact location of the tumor, and she was right. They did a biopsy; the report came back that she had lymphoma. Vianna was right again. Chemotherapy was prescribed, but without medical insurance Vianna could not afford it.

She would not give up. She had a family to feed, her children needed her; she could not die. So, hobbling on crutches, and in constant pain, Vianna continued to see clients. Through it all, she believed God could heal her. She experimented with lemon cleanses, saunas, vitamins and minerals—and prayer.

Ironically, the sicker she grew, the more accurate her readings became. Some weeks later, her aunt came to visit. That night the aunt came down with a stomach flu. The woman moaned and complained and drove Vianna to distraction. In desperation Vianna turned to the technique she used in her readings. "I focused my energy on my crown chakra and sent it into my aunt's body. Then, I commanded God to show me the source of her illness. What I saw was that an E-coli bacteria had lodged in her intestines." Vianna commanded a healing. Suddenly, the pain in her aunt's stomach vanished. Moments later, all the symptoms disappeared. Vianna realized that whatever she had done had worked.

43

The next day, a man came into her office complaining of a severe backache. Vianna tried the same process on him, sending her energy out through her crown chakra into his body; she saw the inflamed muscles and commanded a healing. Instantly, the man's pain disappeared. It had worked again.

Now Vianna began to wonder why she couldn't use the same technique on herself. She repeated the exercise on herself, reaching an ever-deepening state of meditation. She would visualize a ball of light inside her solar plexus and send it three feet, six feet, and higher. Then she commanded "Mother, Father, God, Creator of all that is, I command that my leg be healed and all traces of the cancer gone." And she would see it gone.

She only had to do this once. Vianna's cancerous right leg, which had shrunk three inches shorter than the left, returned to its normal size. Then the swelling subsided, and instantly all of her pain disappeared. Within weeks all her tests came out normal.

Her doctors couldn't figure out what had happened, but Vianna knew she had happened on an important discovery. She began to use the technique on each of her clients. They were getting well; it was working. People, some of them very sick, began to seek her out, flying to Idaho Falls from all over the world. Many of them got well; strangely, others did not.

One day Vianna asked God why she couldn't heal those people. She claimed to have received information about certain genetic defects and how to repair them.

Many healers believe that certain illnesses are karmic and cannot be healed. I hear this over and over, and wonder whether this claim is a cop-out. It gets them off the hook completely, for when healers fail to heal and then explain away their patient's illness as karmic, it is never they who have failed. Yet a part of the claim does seem to make sense. Tibetans explain karma as action. If this is true, then one's ability to heal has to do with one's own actions. And we become a player—if not entirely responsible—in our own healing.

Vianna explained that she had been working in a Theta state. "There are four different frequencies of brain waves: Beta, Alpha, Theta, and Delta. These brain waves are in constant motion. As I am talking and thinking, my mind is in Beta, which has a frequency of 14-28 cycles per second. In an Alpha state, brain waves are at 7-14 cycles per second, which produces a relaxed, meditative state of mind. To understand an Alpha state, close your eyes and imagine a sunset. See in your mind's eye the sun setting against the ocean; sea gulls flying low . . . this is the beginning of an Alpha state.

"A Theta state is a very deep state of relaxation, of perfect calm. It is the state that is used in hypnosis and meditation. Theta brain waves are creative, inspirational, and spiritual. Imagine standing on the top of a mountain and experiencing a total knowing that God is real. Another example is the firewalker in Hawaii. The Kahunas access Theta to walk on hot lava.

45

"In Delta, brain waves are slowed even more and it feels similar to a deep sleep.

"I am convinced that when the Theta state is accessed and one calls upon God, it's like plugging into an electric outlet. It allows you to heal your own body as well as others' using these same techniques. And all aspects of the mind, body, and spirit."

Vianna teaches classes for healers on how to use this technique. She invited me to attend a four-day class she was giving at a conference center in Santa Rosa, California. More than forty healers who had studied her work for the past few years had come to learn the next step in her healing technique.

Vianna sparkles. Dark, curly hair, green eyes, laughing smile. A grandmother at thirty-nine, she looks half her age. Vianna says she's found the strand of DNA that activates youth and vitality. I hope she is right. I can only imagine what she will be able to do if she is right.

Her husband assists in the classes. Each morning, as soon as everyone is seated, he goes around the room and, while kneeling, removes shoes and gently rubs each person's feet with oil of frankincense. I smile, recalling Vianna's story of how they met.

"For years I dreamed of a man that I would be with in the later years of my life. I knew he would have brown hair and blue eyes. I knew he would be either a rancher or a farmer from Montana, and I knew that he would have a child.

"In my dreams I would always call him my guy from Mon-

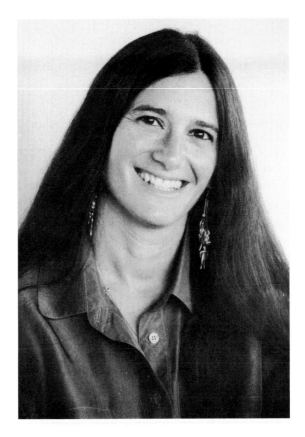

# SANDRA INGERMAN

Sandra Ingerman, a Brooklyn-born woman who now works in
Santa Fe, New Mexico, with clients on spiritual journeying and
soul retrieval. Her training with shamans has led her to believe
that a portion of a person's soul flees during illness and trauma, and
healing occurs only when that portion of the soul returns.

# KATIE
## ENGLEHART

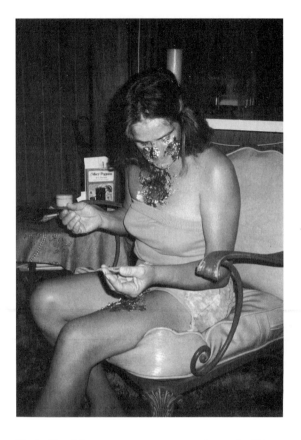

Katie Englehart, a young woman born in Tennessee, is able to
 heal or intuit the ailments of people while in a trancelike state.
Often, moments after entering her trance, goldlike metal
 appears on her face, neck, hands, chest, and back.

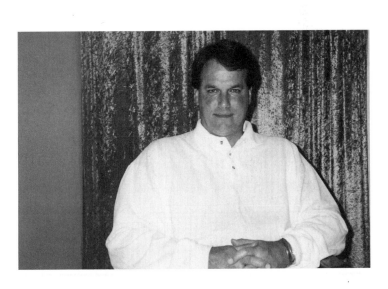

# HOWARD
# WILLS

By the time he was 20 years old, after being visited by a
spirit that allowed him to see through people's bodies
"as if they were made of cellophane," Howard Wills
knew that he wanted to be a healer.

# VIANNA STIBAL

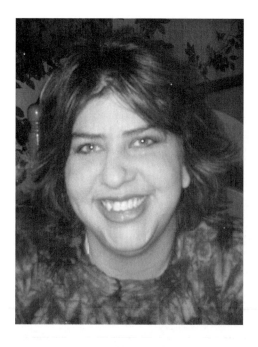

Vianna Stibal, an Idaho housewife, performs "distance healings" over the telephone. She discovered her gift while sketching the faces of coworkers and having flashes of intuition about their health.

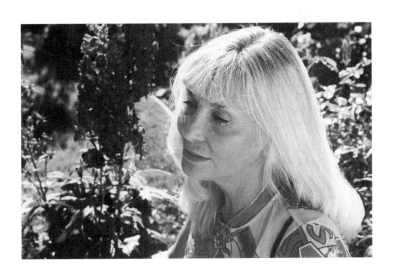

# VIRGINIA
## ELLEN

Virginia Ellen, after a life of pain, exploration, and difficulty,
had a spiritual experience that led her to create
what she calls Sacred Seal Yoga, a practice that has
brought about her own healing and helped many others.

# MILTON
# TRAGER

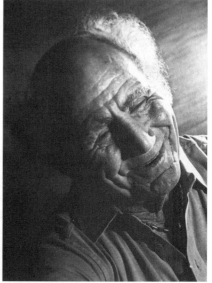

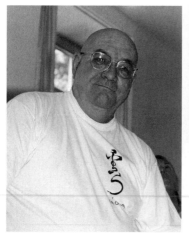

# GARY
# BROWNLEE

Milton Trager developed the Trager Approach, a hands-on
method of healing that had its first success with
victims of polio. Gary Brownlee left his work as an
aerospace engineer to carry on the work of Dr. Trager.

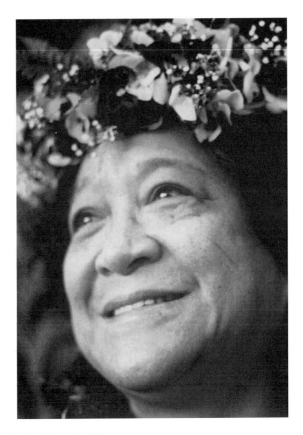

# AUNTIE MARGARET

Auntie Margaret practices the ancient healing art of
lomilomi from her home on the Kona Coast
of the Big Island.

# GERRY
## BOSTOCK

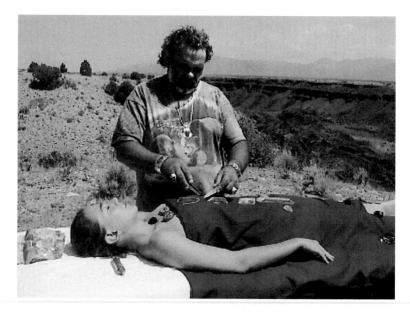

Gerry Bostock, an Australian nicknamed "Bundji" in honor
of his Aboriginal ancestry, learned to heal with
"love, light, crystals, and energy."

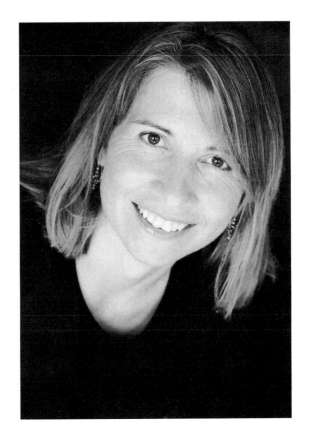

# DR. RUTH
# ZIEMBA

Dr. Ruth Ziemba began her career as a healer as
an oncology nurse and then became a chiropractor.
Her patients claim a healing heat emanates from her hands.

# PETER
## MAXWEL

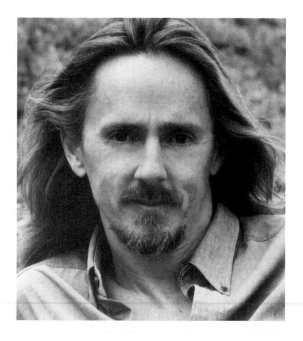

Peter Maxwel, a medal winner for the Australian swim team
in the 1980 and 1984 Olympics, has used
his connection with water to heal other people.

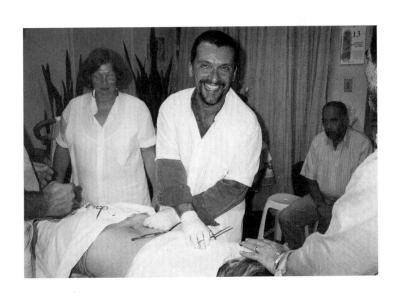

# RUBENS
# FARIA

Rubens Faria is one of the most recent Brazilian mediums
to channel Dr. Fritz, a German military doctor who
died on the battlefield in 1915. Some claim he is
"putting on a show that brings out the best in people."

# JOHN
## OF GOD

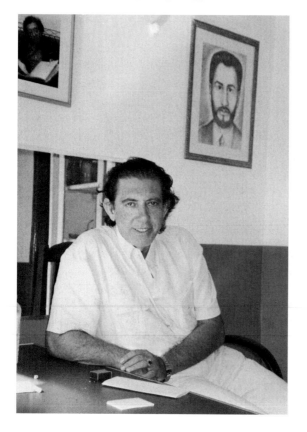

John of God, seated at his desk in front of pictures of two
of the thirty-four entities he channels during his healings.
His center, the Casa de San Inacio, is in Abadiania—
a tiny, remote village in central Brazil, 103 kilometers
from the capital city of Brasilia.

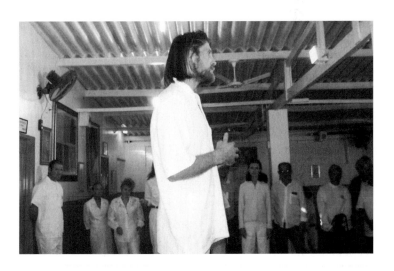

# ULTAN

Ultan, a man who came to the Casa five years ago
from Ireland for healing and never left, instructs those
waiting to meet John of God that they will have the
opportunity to ask for three healings or answers to
questions and that this is a spiritual hospital where one
presents more than their body for healing.

# JOHN OF GOD

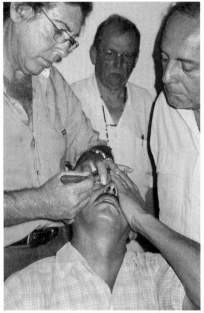

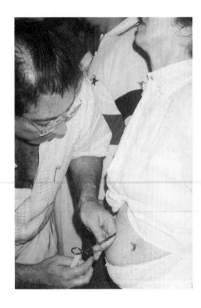

John of God, or Joao de Deus,
     uses a kitchen knife to scrape
     the cornea of a patient.

Hundreds of patients stand in line for surgery at Casa de San
     Inacio and often receive their surgery while in line. Not all
          surgeries are "visible." Many of his patients claim to have
had "invisible operations" performed by spirits.

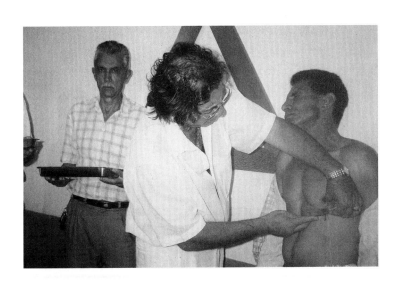

# OR
# JOAO DE DEUS

John of God makes his incisions without the use of
anesthesia. Though he uses unsterilized instruments in his
work, his hospital claims to have never had a single case
of septicemia or infection.

# JOAO-IN-ENTITY

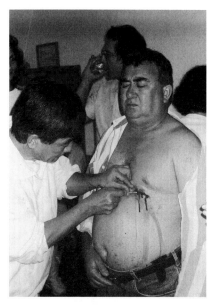

Some surgeries are performed
by Joao's assistants.

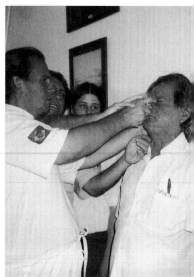

An assistant performs a surgery with the help
of Joao-in-entity.

tana. Time and again I would ask the Creator what his name was, but all I ever got was that he was my guy from Montana.

"In 1997, I met a man. He was both a farmer and a rancher on his parents' land in Montana. He was divorced and had a son. He walked up to me and took my hand and said, "Hello, my name is Guy."

Seated in a large circle around the edge of the room, Vianna calls on one of the women to help demonstrate a practice.

I had noticed the woman earlier. Of all the people present, she seemed the least open. Not unfriendly exactly, but definitely cut off. She appeared to be in her late fifties, stocky, her face half-hidden behind large-framed glasses. Her smile was thin, forced.

Gradually her story unfolded. Her name was Donna. For eight years she was a nun. Married now and studying with Vianna for two years, she had first come to Vianna for her own health problems. Exhausted, bedridden, and depressed, Donna had been through a series of medical doctors: psychiatrists put her on anti-depressants; alternative practitioners prescribed colonics; hypnotherapists tried their magic (none were covered by her insurance). But still she did not get well. Then one day a friend told her about Vianna.

It took three months for Donna to get a telephone appointment with Vianna, but immediately, Vianna saw the cause of Donna's problems: an infection in a root canal was leaking into her system. Vianna pinpointed the exact location of the infected tooth and told Donna that as soon as they got off the phone she

47

was to take a quarter-teaspoon of cream of tartar in a half-cup of water.

The next day Donna went to her dentist and had an X-ray. The tooth was indeed infected, and the infected tooth was precisely where Vianna said it would be.

In subsequent conversations, Vianna discovered Donna had candida. She also had large amounts of mercury and aluminum in her system, a combination that was slowly poisoning her.

Sitting opposite Vianna now in the center of the circle, Donna places her palms on top of Vianna's upturned hands, and eyes closed, they begin.

When each reaches a Theta state, Vianna asks Donna what she is feeling.

"I hate God," Donna says slowly. "I hate God for putting me here."

Vianna waits. After a moment, Donna lets out a cry. She says she can't breathe. She feels she is being strangled. The pain in her neck and upper back is unbearable.

In silence lasting for several minutes, Vianna works on the pain.

Finally, with tears in her voice, Donna says, "No, it isn't God I hate." She takes a deep breath, her chest lifts and she moves her neck with considerably more ease. "It's my life I hate. My mother didn't want me, she already had six children." She went on to describe her sad and troubled life now.

We are witnessing a breakthrough. All these years Donna has been shut down, burying her anger and negativity inside a nun's habit. Color floods Donna's face now and she lets the tears flow.

Exhausted, she went outside to her van and rested a while. When she came back in, I asked her how she felt.

"I wanted to come back in and join the group, but I felt too insecure. I knew everyone would be checking to see if I had changed. Actually, I knew I had reverted back to the usual face I carry: the teacher, the intellectual, the semi-skeptic. It's my protective I.D.

"The message I keep getting is that I have to heal myself, learn the lessons I need so that I can become a more authentic person."

To me, the person I had observed the first day who seemed so tight and shut down was gone without a trace. Donna seemed bright and open now, and maybe on her way to real healing.

Another woman, Sally, tells how she had been diagnosed with malignant melanoma. "It started with a mole on the back of my head. After surgery, several consultations with doctors, and several pathology reviews, they found lesions in my brain.

"They told me there is no treatment for melanoma malignancy that has spread to the brain. Life expectancy is four to six months and can be as short as four weeks. It was right after this news that I heard of Vianna. A family friend had heard of her successes in helping people with serious medical problems and helped us find her.

"Vianna was absolutely wonderful from the start. Even with a heavy schedule she was able to arrange an 'emergency' session with me.

"During this session, she somehow removed the brain lesions. 49 Subsequent brain MRIs have shown that the lesions are gone. A test from the John Wayne Cancer Institute verified that there are no melanoma cells in my blood. This essentially means that after having been diagnosed with this terminal disease, I am now clear of any cancer.

"That wasn't the only thing she did. She told me on my first visit that I had 'pins' in some old root canals that would cause me trouble. Two months later, a massive infection was discovered that resulted from the breakdown of old metal pins inserted during a root canal years ago. After I had brain radiation, I lost my sense of taste, a common side effect. In one of my sessions with Vianna, I mentioned this to her and she made adjustments to the radiation effects and that night I was able to taste again.

"Doctors have not been able to explain these changes. They're completely amazed that my terminal disease simply disappeared. I know the reason: Vianna is truly a miracle maker."

Joel Stock, a chemist in Newark, California, had Parkinson's disease. Vianna suggested one of her liver cleanses of oil and lemon. Within days, he was able to discontinue medication for the tremors, his speech cleared, and he could walk without fear of tripping.

He was also able to discontinue medication that he'd been on for six years since a major heart attack—with, he adds, the consent of his cardiologist. "My heart has been healing, returning to normal. Soon after I started the cleansing process, I had so much energy I wanted to run up and down the stairs in our home. I am far more alert and my ability to focus has greatly improved.

I still have work to do, but I have made dramatic progress . . ."

Typically, healers do not have the resources to follow up on the people they have worked on. So unless the people themselves report back on their progress, there is no way to know if these healings "held." Also, those whose illnesses returned may not wish to stay in contact with the healer.

In Vianna's case, her "soul families" do seem to stay in touch. She reports they are still doing well.

# CHAPTER
# FIVE

# BIG CAT

# HEALER

Who are these people? Were they born with a specific gift? Like a Mozart or an Einstein or a Tiger Woods? Are we all born with the same spark of the divine that can be developed? Many of the healers I interviewed said they developed their gift out of necessity — to heal themselves or a family member. But what exactly was the gift? Will scientists one day discover a "healer" gene?

When I heard about a Chinese healer living in Denver whose healings were said to be so astounding that his identity had to be kept secret lest hordes of people descend on him and the press set up camp outside his door, I had to know more. Could this man hold the key to the gift?

Immediately, I flew to Denver, and promising anonymity, met with the healer and the woman whose child was being treated by him. This is the story that unfolded:

On a quiet residential street in a suburb outside of Denver, a young woman stands waiting at the door of a small house, her gravely ill three-year-old baby boy in her arms. The baby squirms and fusses; the woman shifts him onto her other shoulder and, murmuring softly, strokes his head.

Behind her, a car horn sounds; a couple with a toddler stroll by; a girl with two small white dogs on leashes passes; a delivery truck pulls up to the curb; an old man carrying a plastic grocery bag walks slowly, bent over his cane. It is early spring; tiny pea-green buds dot the trees, red and white geraniums spill over window boxes.

The woman has flown to Denver that morning from her home in Boston to bring her child to the Chinese healer she has heard about. It is her last desperate hope. Her baby had been diagnosed when he was just six months old with a massive growth in the left hemisphere of his brain. A tumor rarely found in an infant and almost always fatal. They operated twice; each time the tumor grew back. The neurosurgeon said the baby could not survive a third operation.

A chiropractor told her about the healer, whom, he warned, was said to be very strict and charged a lot of money.

The woman did not call right away. They had no money; every penny they could scrape together had gone to doctors and hospitals, and they were drowning in debt. But then when the child began to grow weaker and could no longer hold down food, and his fever kept spiking, the woman realized her child would soon die.

Over her husband's protests, she begged and borrowed from family and friends to help her get to Denver.

But now, standing at the door of the healer's house, the woman is terrified. What if the man wants more than they can pay and turns her away? Or what if the man says he can help and gets her hopes up, but he really cannot? She has long ago lost her power to reason. A sob starts in her throat and rises, tears filling her eyes.

The door opens.

The woman blinks back her tears, draws a sharp breath. The man is small and bone-thin. He could be thirty or sixty. Despite his western dress—gray slacks and plaid cotton shirt—he looks like something out of one of those movies where the Chinaman steps out of the shadows brandishing a knife. His hair is tightly pulled back in a ponytail; his skin is the color of rancid butter. But it is the eyes. Small coffee beans in slatted lids, they peer out at her, expressionless.

He bows his head briefly. The baby quickly turns from him, frightened, and buries his head against his mother. The woman forces a smile and extends her hand.

He does not take her hand; instead he bows again, slightly, and says, "Come in, please."

He lets her pass in front of him. "Upstairs, please."

When they reach the top, he reaches in front of her and opens another door. A wail, loud and high-pitched, causes the woman to jump. The child begins to cry.

"Is all right. Not to fear," the man says. He points to a huge tawny cat, the biggest cat the woman had ever set eyes on outside of a zoo, perched right on the top of a couch. Its eyes, an opalescent yellow-green and outlined in black, are fixed on them.

The child grows quiet, awed. "Look, Mommy. Big cat."

"Cat's name Lora," the healer says.

"Hello, Lora," the child says shyly. The healer points to a chair in the middle of the sparsely furnished room.

"You sit, please. Child on lap." The woman sits, places the child so that he can see the cat. She begins to explain about his illness, but the healer shakes his head to silence her. "Not necessary," he says, "I see everything. I see inside head."

He begins his work. Eyes partly closed, trancelike, he stands in front of them and begins to move his hands as if playing a harp, the long, slender fingers quicksilver. Then he stands back a few steps and sweeps his hands up and down, back and forth, with increasing speed and intensity.

Nervously, the woman averts her eyes. She looks at the paintings on the walls: a monstrous tree set against a midnight sky with snakes as branches; a face of an old woman floating in a galaxy surrounded by planets and spaceships.

"Turn baby, please."

The woman turns the child so that he is facing her. His eyes shine bright, so bright she thinks he must be running a fever again. She touches his cheek; it feels normal. She looks up at the healer. "His eyes," she says, pointing to them. "So bright . . . ?"

"Fire coming out," he says. He continues the movements for several minutes. Then he makes a pyramid with his hands above the child's head and holds it there.

Thirty minutes have passed. "You come tomorrow please, same time."

The woman remembers then. "I must ask. What will your fee be?"

"We talk later. Not to worry yourself."

"Do you think you can help him?"

"We will see. Boy may be a little sick tonight. It is natural."

The baby is sick that night. All night. He vomits and has diarrhea and runs a fever. The woman is terrified; she is about to phone the desk to order a taxi to take them to the nearest emergency room, when just as suddenly the fever subsides, and the baby wants to eat. In the morning, the baby points to the foot of the bed.

"Mommy, Lora came to see me."

That afternoon, when she returns to the healer, she tells him about the night before, how sick the child was, and that he dreamed about the cat. "No, no. Not a dream," the healer says. "I send Lora."

He performs the same motions, again for thirty minutes. "Come tomorrow, please. Same time."

57

58

By the third week, the baby begins to gain weight. He has stopped vomiting, his eyes are brighter, more focused, and he's talking a blue streak. The dizzy spells are all but gone.

On the last day, the woman takes out her checkbook. The healer bows. "No. Not necessary." She tries to thank him, but he will accept no gratitude. As they are about to leave, the child suddenly reaches out his arms to the healer. For the first time, the woman sees him smile.

When they get back to Boston, she tells the doctor about the healer and asks him to do another CT scan. The woman is devastated: The scan shows the tumor is still there, perhaps a bit smaller, but definitely there.

Her husband rolls his eyes, shrugs.

That night the woman calls the healer. "No, no," he says. "Is not tumor, only dead tissue. Get PET scan. They will see."

The woman requests a PET scan. The healer was right.

Three months later, the tumor still has not returned. The child is stronger and healthier. Some mornings the baby tells his mother, "Lora came to see me last night. She sat there," he says, pointing to the foot of his bed. Seven years later, the little boy attends school, plays with friends, and sometimes remembers Lora, the big cat who made him well. Doctors could never explain why the tumor did not reappear. Yet, the neurosurgeon in charge of the child's case refused to acknowledge that the child had been "healed" by the Chinaman, saying only, "Whatever the guy did probably didn't hurt."

But a year later, a well-known actor suffering a recurrence of lung cancer also found his way to that same Chinese healer. Full of hope, needing to believe, and dreading another round of chemotherapy that would cost him a role in a coming movie, the actor spent several weeks—and many thousands of dollars— under the healer's care. As the days went by and the actor's condition worsened, the healer cautioned him not to rush treatments. "More time, more time," he said until there was no more time.

Ironically, of all the many newspapers that reported the actor's death, only one tabloid told the true story.

# CHAPTER
# SIX

# SACRED

# SEALS

## VIRGINIA ELLEN

When Bill, my agent, asked me to drive down for lunch at a restaurant near his office to meet a healer from Idaho, I expected to meet another gifted housewife. What I did not expect was a tall, blond, former fashion model in her fifties.

At first I thought the attractive woman at the table was a friend of Bill's and that the healer would be along soon. When it became clear that Virginia Ellen was the healer I had been brought to meet, I forced myself to look away from her perfectly French-manicured fingernails and expensive-looking jewelry to her eyes. Robin's egg blue, they radiated warmth and a depth inconsistent with the rest of her image. Healers do not have to be plain, I reminded myself, anymore than they have to be poor.

After lunch, we went back to Bill's house and sat in his garden. Virginia offered to give us a demonstration of her chakra activation technique. Willing subjects, we followed her instructions.

Placing both hands over her solar plexus, asking us to do the same, she took several breaths. Then in a high-pitched tone that frightened the birds out of nearby trees, Virginia made the Om sound. We joined in. Three times in a row. The high tones connect us with God energy, Virginia explained, so that healing can occur.

Another exercise had us connecting with the first chakra, the seat of passion power, and saying, emphatically, "I can, I know I can."

She told me about her yoga practice, which she has named Sacred Seal Yoga, and the healings the practice has brought about. And she told of her journey from the edge of despair.

We made a date to continue our conversation at the home of a friend where she would be stopping on her way back to Idaho. Wondering if I had uncovered a hotbed of healers in the potato state, I asked her if she knew of Vianna. She didn't. Virginia is a recent transplant from California, where she had lived during her married years.

She was born in New York City's Lower East Side in 1943 into a life of poverty. For the first five years of her life, her family was on welfare. Virginia's world was one of street violence, gangs who beat people with socks filled with dirt, the paddy wagon that pulled up every night on gambling raids. Sexually molested at six, she lived in constant fear.

When Virginia was eight, her father got a job with Hughes Aircraft and moved the family to Long Beach, California. But by then Virginia had shut down. Her strict Catholic family reinforced her fears. At seventeen, she married her brother's friend. They had a daughter and, eighteen months later, a son. After the birth of her son, doctors found tumors in her uterus and performed a hysterectomy.

At six months, she noticed that sunlight bothered her baby boy and that he seemed excessively fussy. Then he began to vomit every morning. The pediatrician thought it might be some sort of virus, but another doctor diagnosed a brain tumor. Nine months later, after six surgeries and radiation, the baby died.

When a priest assured her it was "God's will," Virginia, wondering what kind of God could allow such a thing to happen, stopped going to church.

Angry, depressed, crying constantly, she tried psychiatric therapy, took anti-depressants, and finally, a year later, she threw herself into the country club life made possible by her husband's high-paying job. She played tennis every day, joined the Junior League, and modeled for charity events. That led to an interest in the fashion world, where she eventually built a successful business. A year later, she and her husband adopted a four-day-old baby boy.

From the outside, the beautiful Virginia seemed to have found the perfect life — Cadillac, big house with a swimming pool. But with it all, she had "an overwhelming, suffocating, lack of self-esteem."

Men were attracted to her and she yearned for romance. She wanted a divorce. But her freedom would cost her the house, the swimming pool, the Cadillac, and all financial security. So Virginia set out on a spiritual shopping spree — from est training to Science of Mind, to a cultlike spiritual community in Washington State. She followed gurus and read books on spirituality,

63

but in none of these things did she find an answer to her questions or her feelings of emptiness. She felt as if she was sliding backward, back to the poverty and fear of her youth.

One night, awake at four in the morning with a raging fever and severe stomach flu, she laid alone and delirious. "I'm dying," she thought. "I've never been happy, and now I'm dying." She felt herself drift out of her body into a peaceful light. Out of that light a figure appeared and told her she must agree to change every concept of her life. That figure, she believed, was Jesus.

She doesn't remember how long that lasted. But later, Virginia woke up recovered and spiritually renewed. She finally understood the reason for the years of tragedy and failure. She began to receive clairaudient instructions on how to live her life, what foods to eat, and what foods to avoid. All this, she understood, was to prepare her for the teachings that would allow her to become a healer and a teacher. Come spring she would begin to channel Jesus and he would teach her how to heal and teach. She understood that she had chosen to experience the tragedy of death and fear and poverty to learn the compassion necessary to become an effective healer.

Over the coming months, again and again, Virginia would ask herself, "Am I making all this up?"

Yet she could feel her life expanding. In meditation, she would hear a voice instructing her, "Be quiet, I can hear you. I can hear what you're feeling when I'm working with you." Gradually, Virginia came to understand the channeling she was receiving and merged it with her own practice of yoga and meditation. Soon her seven-day Sacred Seals retreats were filling up with earnest students.

In class, many students reported seeing a gold light around her.

As Virginia's clients heard of my interest in her work, many wrote to share with me stories of their experiences with her.

Lou Fleming was one. He had been suffering with Chronic Fatigue Syndrome for years. His condition had steadily worsened until he felt near death. He had lost more than fifty pounds in five years and could no longer get out of bed. His team of doctors, both Western and alternative, had nothing more to offer in the way of treatment. His hope had vanished; he was ready to give up. Then, he found his way to Virginia.

"Virginia was able to merge her energy and her consciousness with mine, and with a specific body part or symptom, she can hear the consciousness of that symptom speak. She told me that in order to heal the emotional pain, I first had to feel it."

She took Lou through a series of affirmations, replacing his belief that he didn't want to live with new beliefs. "I choose to live, thank you God for restoring my health." Over and over, loudly, as if he meant it.

"What came next was a complete surprise. I noticed a few minutes afterward that I was feeling less nausea than I had felt in a long time. Then I became aware that it was taking less effort to move about the room, I had more energy than I had before."

Since then, Lou's healing has steadily improved. He calls it a work in progress.

As with so many of the healers I had been meeting, Virginia had walked through fire. Out of the embers a spark was ignited, and Virginia emerged a healer.

# CHAPTER
## SEVEN

# HOOKING-UP

## MILTON TRAGER
## AND GARY BROWNLEE

I was beginning to notice a pattern. Many of the healers I had met had stumbled upon their gift while they were doing something else—like a person who walks along a beach and notices some sparkly thing in the sand, a beautiful piece of sea glass, perhaps, or a shell that feels magical in the hand.

Gary Brownlee was busy building spacecraft when he happened across the thing that would change his life. For more than twenty years he had been working as an aerospace engineer on such projects for NASA as the *Saturn V* rocket used in the Apollo missions, then on the *Viking* spacecraft that landed on Mars, and the *Voyager* spacecraft that took the photographs of Jupiter, Saturn, and Uranus. Until the day in 1975 when a friend suggested that he go to Big Sur in California for a week at the Esalen Institute.

Gary had been through a rough divorce, and his work in the aerospace industry had become increasingly stressful. A week on the wild and rocky coast of Northern California sounded good. One of the workshops offered massage training, which he took to enthusiastically. He discovered then that he had "hands." He stayed on another week, learning and exchanging sessions, discovering more about the structure of the human body. As soon as he got home, he went into the garage and built a massage table and got his friends to let him work on them.

Meanwhile, every other aspect of his life had grown so stressful that his hair was beginning to fall out in clumps, a sign that the time had come to turn his life in another direction. Gary decided to take a two-month leave of absence from his work to think about what he wanted to do. During this time he went back to Esalen to do a training in Trager Psychophysical Integration, which was later renamed the Trager Approach.

Dr. Milton Trager had developed an "approach," as he called it, to treat people with various neuro-muscular disorders—from Parkinson's to muscular dystrophy to acute back problems to people who were simply seeking to improve their body awareness. He watched as Trager, in a state of what he called "active meditation," made a deep connection with the person whose body he was working on. Trager called this *hooking-up*.

"Hook-up is like the measles," Trager explained. "You catch it from someone who's got it. I want you all to experience your mind asking, 'Well, how free is that?' Pause a moment, come deeper into this state, and ask yourself again: 'Well, what is freer than that?' Every moment of every session . . . just you and this feeling going hand in hand. Take them to this state, take them, take them, bring them along, give them something more so that they can be different."

Gary knew then and there what he wanted to do with his life. "That experience had taken me from outer space to inner space."

He could see the parallels: The body is a structure held together with living bone that is pliable—"Not dried-out like a chicken wishbone"—and muscle that is elastic and can be manipulated and re-educated. "Principles I used as a structural analyst in the aerospace industry—weight, leverage, vibration, impulse and momentum, and frequency—applied to the work Trager was doing. The hardest thing is to get a spacecraft out of the gravitational pull," Gary says. "So it is with the human body, to re-educate muscles, postural habits, tissue, behavioral patterns that keep the body tense and compressed."

Gary learned quickly. For the next few years, he worked only part-time (he was then a consultant on communications satellites at Hughes) and spent every spare moment in training with Dr. Trager. Finally, he left completely to build his own practice. Eventually, Gary became the first man authorized by Dr. Trager to teach his method.

I met Gary at the physical therapy studio where I go to work out on Pilates machines. My instructor, Dianne Khebreh, knew of my interest in alternative healing methods and suggested I meet Gary.

69

He is huge. With his bald head and massive body, he looks like Mr. Clean. I follow him into one of the massage rooms and lie face-up, fully clothed, on the table.

He begins by taking my head in his hands and gently rolling it back and forth from one hand to the other, until my neck releases. Then, with gentle pressure, he pushes my shoulders down, stretching the muscles. "You don't have to do anything," he says. "Don't even try to relax. I'll do that for you."

He gives my head a tug. I feel warmth creep all the way down my spine to my tailbone. Then he takes my arms and legs through a series of large movements to find my range of motion. "The goal," he says, "is not to try. Trying is effort and effort creates tension. What Trager does is to effect change in the unconscious mind with a different feeling experience of the muscle structure."

Then gently—always gently—he shakes each leg, each arm, jiggling the muscles and joints free.

He tells me to turn over onto to my stomach and begins to rock my body from side to side, loosening, letting go. I am floating. I am free. I am released from the earth's pull.

Gary tells me my body will remember this feeling, that I can recall it any time I wish and my body will respond. I will be able to create my own mini-session.

Milton Trager, born in 1908, became an M.D. late in life, at the age of forty-two, and lived a long, full, and incredibly productive life until his death in 1997. Before medical school, Trager worked as a lay practitioner, using his technique with astounding success with polio victims and others with crippling conditions. When he became an M.D., Trager incorporated his hands-on approach into his practice of general medicine and physical rehabilitation.

In 1975, Dr. Trager was invited to demonstrate his work at the Esalen Institute. From that workshop a large following formed. Two years later, Dr. Trager closed his private medical practice to devote his time to his growing number of students.

One statistic that impressed me indicated his success in treating back pain: Out of over 5,000 painful lower backs that he has treated in fifty-five years, ninety percent of the patients claimed to have had "notable *and lasting* relief."

"Lasting" is the operative word here. Unlike many healers, Dr. Trager, because he was trained as an M.D., kept medical records that tracked the results of his care with his patients.

In 1958, Trager studied with the Maharishi Mahesh Yogi, who said to him, "It is natural for the mind to want to go to the field of greater happiness, towards deeper understanding, towards expansiveness, towards connecting with the sources of our being."

Milton Trager had found a sensory means of redirecting the footsteps of someone who has lost the way.

Dr. Trager wrote: "My work is directed towards reaching the unconscious mind of the client. Every move, every thought, communicates how the tissue should feel when everything is right. The mind is the whole thing . . . I am convinced that for every physical nonyielding condition, there is a psychic counterpart in the unconscious mind, corresponding exactly to the

71

degree of the physical manifestation. Trager consists of the use of the hands to influence deep-seated psycho-physiological patterns in the mind and to interrupt their projection into the body's tissues. These patterns often develop in response to adverse circumstances such as accidents, surgery, illness, poor posture, emotional trauma, stresses of daily living, or poor movement habits. The purpose of my work is to break up these sensory and mental patterns which inhibit free movement and cause pain and disruption of normal function. My approach is to impart to the client what it is like to feel right in the sense of a functionally integrated body-mind. Since the inhibiting patterns are affected at the source—the mind—the client can experience long-lasting benefits. The result is general functional improvement."

Today, Dr. Trager's work is being carried on by more than fifteen hundred teacher-practitioners in the U.S. and in other countries around the world.

One Trager practitioner, Royce Ann Heard, tells about her first experience with the work. She had suffered for years from back pain due to scoliosis. Her head and upper torso were noticeably bent to the right and her breath was constricted. By fourteen, she had had three spinal fusion surgeries and had come to accept that she would live with acute pain for the rest of her life.

During the first few months of Trager sessions, while her bones and muscles began to shift from their longtime position, she still had pain. But soon she could tell the difference between the pain of improvement and the old pain.

As her body changed, so did her self-esteem. She left her career as a math teacher to become a Trager practitioner.

"My body continues to change even after fifteen years of sessions. Each new session reinforces and deepens what my body has learned and takes it yet another step forward . . ."

I have two more sessions, one with Dianne Khebreh, the woman with whom I do my Pilates workout who is also a Trager practitioner. The other session is with Ninfa Bramble, a physical therapist aide who works part-time at the studio.

Afterward, I notice that my walk is freer, easier, and my posture is better without my consciously correcting back and shoulders. And when next I go back to work out on the Pilates machines, I feel like the girl on the flying trapeze.

No evidence of the placebo effect here.

# CHAPTER
# EIGHT

# LAND OF
# LOMILOMI

## AUNTIE MARGARET

In a place that closely resembles paradise, on the Kona Coast of the Big Island, lives an eighty-six-year-old Hawaiian Kahuna affectionately known as "Auntie" Margaret Machado, described by many as the Island's most highly esteemed Kahuna *lomilomi* teacher and practitioner.

Kahuna, as defined in a Hawaiian dictionary, is a priest, sorcerer, magician, wizard, or minister (whether male or female) and is used as a title, like M.D. or Ph.D. A Kahuna is a master of a craft, such as Hawaiian herbs, *lomilomi*, canoe carving, long distance sea navigation, agriculture. *Lomilomi* is an ancient art of spiritual, mental, and physical bodywork, passed down in families from a master.

Orphaned at four by her mother's death and raised at the Mis-

75

sionary Home on Oahu, it was her Big Island grandfather, John Ahaulakeali'i, a Kahuna priest of the *alii* or royalty class who named Margaret at birth for the work she would do. He chanted over her just before he died, when she was ten years old, and is said to have given her his gift at that time.

Nicknamed *Ko'o*, which means "very strong," her grandfather was skilled in *ho'ponopono,* meaning "to set things right"—the art of mental cleansing by the use of discussion, examination, and prayer. He chose her at birth as the one to whom he would pass on his knowledge. "My grandfather leaned over and breathed on me four times—once on each cheek, my forehead, and the top of my head. Then he chanted in Hawaiian. He had given me the blessing and my Hawaiian name, which in English means 'The flower that sees through to your soul.'"

After finishing high school, Margaret became a practical nurse, worked as a masseuse for sports teams, cut hair, grew herbs, played the organ in church, even prepared the dead for burial—until she met and married "Uncle Dan" and had four children. In her spare time, she made leis out of the seeds and shells that Daniel, a fisherman, gathered each day, drilling tiny holes in them to make leis. At first, Margaret gave the leis away to tourists, but later she and the children sold them at a little stand at Kealakekua Bay. They sold enough leis to put all four children through college.

Auntie Margaret had been giving *lomilomi* only to family members, but over the years people began to come to her begging for massage and herbs and eventually to learn what she knew. She became the first person to share the art of *lomilomi* outside the Hawaiian culture—against her family's wishes.

I have flown to the Big Island from Maui with my friend, Mollie, who I was visiting. We rent a car and after an interminable, frustrating series of wrong turns, we find our way to Auntie Margaret's house. Later on, whenever I refer to that maddening drive, her students laugh. Apparently, finding her is all part of the initiation rite.

She is small, just a little over five feet, and sturdy. She greets us with open arms. "Do you need a hug?" she asks. "You know, God only sends me people I can help."

She introduces us to Uncle Dan, who sits at his desk. Auntie Margaret buzzes around fetching photographs to show us and filling us in on her family history. One photo shows her on the beach with her three young daughters; another is of her son; yet another is of her eldest daughter, Nerita, who was a nurse in California before she returned home to Hawaii to help her mother. Nerita, she explains, now teaches classes to students who come from every corner of the world to learn *lomilomi*.

We ask if *lomilomi* is anything like a Swedish massage; Auntie Margaret emphatically says, "No. *Lomilomi* is very different. It's a tender, loving touch. You must pray from the heart, empty the mind, and let the Lord take over and heal. Your hand has to be relaxed and gentle, because behind every stroke is a reason. You have to find the rhythm, the breath, the beat

77

of the heart, the flow of spinal fluid. Like the Hulu dance."

She explains the Hawaiian word *lomilomi* means "going to and from." "To work in and out, as the claws of a contented cat. An authentic *lomilomi* treatment goes far beyond massage," she says. "It is meant to heal mind, body, and spirit with assistance from the divine."

She resists the title Kahuna ("I am just Auntie Margaret") and says she is not the healer; all healing comes from God. "I am his instrument. My grandfather was a Christian and a praying man who practiced *ho'ponopono*." Although methods varied from family to family, it was the village Kahuna who over a period of years would train the family member who was destined to inherit this knowledge (as Auntie Margaret's grandfather did). This long training period would ensure the trainee's ability and vocation as a *lomilomi* healer.

The treatment is a combination of prayer, body manipulation, energy work, massage, and Hawaiian herbs. "Mana" (life force) is transferred directly from the healer into the patient.

Auntie Margaret turns to me and asks that I remove my glasses, earrings, and the beads I am wearing. She wants me to get up onto the table so she can have a look at me. Placing her hands on my legs, my chest, and on the top of my head, she muses aloud, "We are beautifully made . . ."

Then she takes my bare foot in her hands. "My, you were stubborn when you were a teenager, weren't you?" Takes my other foot and examines my toes, bending them backward and forward. "Don't worry. Now you're a nice girl." She looks at my fingers, and says, "You were very sick a few years ago, but you're fine now."

I ask her what she sees in the toes and fingers.

"I read the way the toes bend. How your feet have grown tells me how your bones developed. Same with the fingers. And the muscles in your face. If one side of the face pulls, the carotid artery is tight. That affects the heart. A person would have to change their diet and take more exercise. Your face tells all about you. I always tell my students, 'Your countenance will show against you!'

"Always remember to look at your heart each day when the sun goes down. And to forgive yourself, your family, and friends. You must empty your heart of any bad feelings. Red cells build when you're happy."

Then Auntie Margaret puts Mollie on the table and observes that she has had problems with her hip. She gives her a series of exercises to do.

Ten miles down a long hill along a bumpy road is a small, weathered beach cottage. It is Auntie Margaret's school. The coastline is dramatic: waves slap against black lava rocks, a small boat is tied to a launch, and just beyond is a tiny sandy beach. A mile out in the bay is the Captain Cook monument where dolphins come to play.

I am told this place has long been regarded as a spiritual center and a source of powerful energy. Students come from around the world for a month-long course in the technique of *lomilomi* massage and cleansing. Classes are given in physiology and anatomy by Mark Lamore, Doctor of Oriental Medicine.

As many as nineteen students at a time come from every part of the world, from captains of industry and movie stars to massage therapists and surfers. They sleep on the lanai in tents and in the open hut in back, and for one month they live as a community, a family.

Dr. Lamore gives me a detailed outline of the day's activities for the ten-day cleansing program: The day begins at six with a sixty-five ounce drink of seawater mixed with fresh water. This acts as a cathartic and begins the cleansing process.

[*Note:* at this point I am issued a warning, which I pass along to the reader: The description that follows is not for the faint of heart or queasy of stomach.]

Each person is given a five-gallon bucket that becomes his or her personal toilet during the "cleanse." For two or three days during the cleanse, everyone brings his or her bucket to the hut in back for inspection. Auntie's husband, Uncle Dan, has been known to toss an old penny into someone's bucket as a prank, or a handful of macadamia nuts. From time to time, Auntie Margaret puts on her surgical gloves and inspects the contents of each bucket. She looks for worms, parasites, and other irregularities. A special "formula," taken three times a day, contains grape juice, herbs, and fiber as well as bentonite and clay powder that draws out toxins and acts as a bulking agent. This firms the feces in such a way that it provides a mirror image of the construction of the colon, "like a Jell-O mold," Dr. Lamore says. "She can see polyps or irregularities in the diverticula—pouches or sacs—much as doctors see with a colonoscopy."

Dr. Lamore explains that the colon is the body's sewer pipe, where years of sludge can build up and clog the system, causing a host of illnesses.

In the afternoon, students rest, take steam baths, and swim out to where the dolphins play. Evenings are spent playing music and writing in the journals they are encouraged to keep.

Then they sit in a circle for "talk-story time," an island term for talking about themselves and their problems: a spiritual and mental cleansing.

Dr. Mark Lamore tells the story of a surfer, a young man in his early thirties, who appeared one day asking for help. He had been diagnosed with lymphoma. He stayed the full month, followed the cleansing program, and then went home to Kauai. No one heard from him again until five years later when he drove up to the cottage with his wife and children.

Another staff member, Mimi George, a doctor of cultural anthropology and an advanced *lomilomi* practitioner as well as leader of cleanses, told me about a remarkable woman, a student of Auntie Margaret's, Glenna Wilde.

Glenna was working her way through naturopathic medical school doing landscaping. Her final assignment before leaving the job was to clear a field of dandelions. She tried to convince the people who had hired her that dandelions were a medicinal plant and should not be destroyed, but they insisted. Glenna needed the money to get her through her final year of medical school, so she did the work.

She loaded a barrelful of herbicide onto the back of her pickup. As she drove a freak wind came up and blew the powder onto her body. She became seriously ill with herbicide poisoning. Her weight dropped to ninety-three pounds, her color took on a greenish hue, and she grew weaker by the day. Glenna went from one specialist to another, but none of them seemed to know how to get the poison out of her body.

81

Four years earlier, while on a break from medical school,
Glenna had studied with Auntie Margaret. When she found she
was not getting well, Glenna phoned Auntie Margaret, who told
her to come as soon as she could.

Glenna put up her tent close to the porch. By then she was so
weak she had to crawl out on her hands and knees five times a
day to take the formula.

On the eighth day, Glenna felt strong enough to walk. She
started down the beach path but had to stop and dig a hole to
use as an emergency toilet. She passed brown-green and yellow
slime that looked and smelled exactly like the poison. She had
finally flushed it out of her system.

After another six cleanses, Glenna was well. She went back to
medical school and got her degree in naturopathic medicine and
for the next few years had a thriving practice in Kauai and Alaska.

In 1998, when she moved to Auntie's, Glenna, who loved to
swim, was coming back along the beach path when she stumbled
and fell on a lava rock. The bone on her lower leg was cracked;
the pain was terrible. When she returned from the emergency
room with an X-ray showing a crack in her bone, Auntie Margaret put Glenna on the table and put her hands on the broken
area and said the Lord's Prayer. Glenna saw something others had
reported seeing: Auntie's eyes had turned red during the session.

When she took her hands away, Glenna's leg tingled. And
when she looked, she saw tiny rainbows along the fracture.
Glenna slept for an hour. When she awoke, the pain had disappeared and she could walk without her crutches. A week later,

Glenna had another X-ray. All signs of the fracture were gone.

But her kidneys had been so damaged by the earlier poisoning that she needed a transplant. Yet her system could not tolerate the immune-suppressing drugs she needed to take afterward to aid her body's acceptance of the new kidneys. Seven-and-a-half years after her kidney transplant, Glenna passed away.

A service was held at the beach, with Auntie Margaret officiating. Her friends went out in canoes to spread her ashes where Glenna liked to swim. According to Mimi, the dolphins put on quite a show.

As Mimi tells it, Auntie Margaret had given Glenna sixteen years—valuable years as a teacher and practitioner of advanced *lomilomi* and leader of cleanses.

In the late 80s, Auntie Margaret suffered an accident. She was disembarking from a plane, returning home to the Big Island from a trip, and happened to be the last one off the small prop jet. While she was still on the tarmac, the airplane turned and the blast from the engine knocked her down and blew her some thirty feet. She suffered fractures in both knees and had to have five lumbar vertebrae fused.

Although she lives with constant pain, somehow she still supervises the classes. Over the years, Auntie Margaret has taught thousands of students and touched many thousands of people. "You never get tired when you have love in your heart," she says.

# CHAPTER NINE

# AT THE

# VOICE FARM

## WARREN BARIGIAN

Why would Meat Loaf, the famous rock singer, fall during a performance, injure his knee, and not be able to sing? Of all the best doctors, chiropractors, acupuncturists, hypnotists, herbalists, and psychiatrists, none could give Meat Loaf his voice back. Not for three years could the famous rock star sing a note. Then, three years later, someone told him about voice coach and healer Warren Barigian. After seven sessions, Meat Loaf was back in the recording studio.

And how is it that another pop singer with a serious drug problem that persisted after two lengthy stays in rehab stopped cold turkey after three sessions and is still clean six years later?

Warren Barigian had been a voice coach to professional singers for five or six years when he accidentally discovered that in using his technique to retrain the voice, spontaneous healing occurred on many levels. Following that discovery, he decided to take a year to study anatomy, the respiratory system, brain chemistry—anything that could explain what he was now convinced to be so: that the voice was a gateway to the breath, the brain, and healing on many levels.

I drive up to Yosemite to try to find out what Warren is doing. His home, on four acres in the Yosemite Valley, is a few miles from the entrance to one of America's great national parks and in full view of the pine-blanketed Sierras.

The house is lodge-like, with cozy pine-paneled rooms filled with overstuffed couches, brick fireplaces, a wood-burning stove, and a loft with several bedrooms. Warren explains that he often holds seminars for as many as twenty people.

Warren is a burly bear of a man in his sixties, with halo of bright white hair, a powerful voice, and a booming laugh. He welcomes students and visitors alike with a hug and then heads straight for the kitchen.

Warren's second great passion is cooking. He introduces me to Joe, a student, who stands at the sink rinsing salad greens. Here everyone is considered family. Joe has flown in from Holland, where he is currently living, for two-a-day sessions—one in the morning, another in the evening.

A composer and singer, Joe first studied with Warren seven

years before, when he was living in San Francisco. These days he divides his time between South America and Holland.

He first came to Warren to work on improving his singing voice, but after a few sessions he noticed some marked changes in the way he felt about himself and his way of being in the world. Ridden with anxiety most of his adult life, resulting in a string of bad relationships that always ended in ruin, Joe was failing rapidly in both his personal and professional life. All that changed. "Four or five sessions were like five years of therapy," he tells me.

"Why? What does he do?" I ask.

Joe agrees to allow me to observe his evening session. In the studio, just off the living room, is a massage table. Two leather-padded chairs are perpendicular to each other, a wall of books and tapes is nearby, and a strange assortment of equipment that looks as if it belongs in an auto mechanic's shop is placed near the chairs. Warren explains these are the tools he uses to break through energy blocks on certain points on the shoulder, along the leg and thigh, and on the solar plexus.

Joe sits in one chair; Warren takes the other. I watch from a corner of the couch.

"There is so much information in the voice. Every facet of your life is imprinted in the way you speak," Warren explains. "As children, our very survival depended on how we adapted to our surroundings, whether hostile or benign. To an infant, a delay of a few minutes between crying and being fed could be

87

felt as life threatening. That could lead to deep-seated adaptive

behavior. From a purely energetic viewpoint, that adaptation is always negative because it limits our options as adults."

The session begins. Joe takes a few full breaths, followed by a series of rapid ones. Warren has him make the "aaah" sound, then an extended "eeeh," each in varying pitches, repeating Warren's sounds. Then with one hand on Joe's shoulder, the other on his head, Warren guides Joe into a rocking motion, back and forth and sideways. This continues for several minutes.

At the height of one of the breaths, Warren commands, "Hold and compress, hold it . . ." Then louder and with more intensity he says, "Lean back now, hold onto it." Joe's eyes are closed; his face is flushed red. Moments pass, perhaps only ten seconds, then Joe slowly releases the breath and opens his eyes. He looks dazed, eyes wide, unseeing.

Warren turns to me and explains. "That was a paraconscious state Joe was in." I want to ask what that is exactly, but Warren has already begun to use one of the noisy machines, the one that looks like a car buffer.

Joe's eyes focus on me. I give him a small, relieved smile. Draping a towel over Joe's leg, Warren runs the machine up and down along the fibula bone where, Warren says, emotions are stored from early childhood. "The timeline," he says.

It sounds like something between a buzz saw and a jack-hammer. Joe jumps a bit and winces. I sink deeper into the couch. I have no idea what is happening here, but I am not sure I would want it happening to me.

"Under stress," Warren is explaining, "the key sources of bio-peptides, such as the thymus gland, upper and lower gut, outer thighs and ankles, can bypass the blood/brain barrier and enter emotional receptors in the brain. The use of vibration and pressure releases these peptides into the bloodstream, so that they can travel freely to the brain. The mental gaps created by the stress conditions then become filled by new molecules open for positive training."

I have no idea what any of that means. I tell him so, and Warren assures me I will soon understand.

The session ends with Joe making a series of sounds that are certainly deeper and fuller than before. And he looks utterly happy and relaxed.

Over dinner, Warren asks Joe to tell me what he was feeling during the session. Joe answers carefully, trying to recreate the moment. "For several seconds—I can't tell how long—I'm out. Not passed out, but certainly in some altered state. When I return to full consciousness, I am aware that I am seated in a room and that there is a large, kindly man supporting me. For just a moment I'm not sure where I am or who the man is exactly. The room seems to be shaking. As it settles down, my body movements slow, and then I am aware of where I am, who I am with, and what I am doing. My body is warm, and I feel very alive and energized. When I speak, my voice now is deeper and more resonant."

I agree. The timbre of his voice is still different. Not husky, as if it's been strained, just fuller and very pleasant.

"It's like I've made a ten-second visit to heaven," Joe says. "I can almost remember dream-like images; they're there on the tip of my mind, but too elusive to bring back."

"Does this blanking-out thing happen every session?" I ask.

An ancient toy poodle named Me Too comes to the table looking for a handout. Joe picks her up and sits her on his lap. Warren is in the kitchen getting the salad.

"No, but sometimes it'll happen five or ten times during a forty-five or fifty-minute session."

"Were you ever frightened?"

Joe smiles. "Never. This man's a genius. I started coming to Warren to improve my singing voice, and that was a tremendous success.

"More than that though, I've become less irritable and anxious than before. I'm more sensitive to what I'm feeling in my body."

"In what ways?" I ask. I still cannot get a handle on how it works.

"I feel radiant energy in my legs that I've never felt before, the muscles in my face and jaw are more relaxed, and I breathe more freely. I laugh more easily, my sense of humor has drastically improved," Joe adds with a sardonic smile.

"I have become more aware of my surroundings and more present in my relationships instead of always analyzing everything like I used to."

Warren has gone outside to collect eggs for the morning.

"Did you tell him what your problems were in the beginning—what you were looking to change in yourself?" I ask.

"That's the weirdest thing. I didn't have to. He seemed to know just by listening to my ordinary speaking voice. I don't know how he does it, but I am constantly surprised by the changes in my perception and in my behavior each passing day since I began working with Warren."

That evening, after one of Warren's memorable dinners, we settle in the living room. I am curious to know more about him.

Warren grew up on his parents' farm in Fresno, California. They were hardworking people of Turkish and Greek descent. After school and every summer Warren worked alongside his father.

At Fresno State College he majored in education. After a six-month stint in the Army Reserves, Warren moved to L.A. to study voice. He loved to sing and hoped his powerful baritone-bass voice might lead to a professional career in opera. Meanwhile, he taught school, first in the L.A. school system; then as he got more private students, he began to teach voice full time. People's voices had always interested him. He could always hear the emotion—repression, fear, or lack of authenticity—behind the sound.

He first began to loosen the muscles he sensed were blocking the free flow of energy to the throat with his strong hands. (Warren had played football in college.) After a while, his students began to report profound changes, not only in their voices,

91

but also in their overall energy. Some even reported an unexplained, sudden disappearance of whatever symptom, physical or psychological, they were dealing with at the time.

One day, while working with a male student in his early thirties, something happened that changed the course of Warren's work. He had been applying pressure to certain trigger points on the student's neck and shoulder to open his breathing, then Warren sat down at the piano and had the student make a series of sounds along with the notes he struck.

He got up from the piano to reposition the student. Then, placing one hand on the student's abdomen, and the other on his middle back, he had him take a deep breath. At the top of his breath, he told him to force out the "aaah" sound.

Suddenly, the student began to lose his balance. He leaned against the piano, color drained from his face, and looked as if he might pass out. Warren was terrified. He didn't know what he had done to cause such a reaction.

A few seconds later, the student responded. When he spoke, to their amazement, it was with a new voice. The following week, the student reported that he felt stronger and more energetic and that his voice had remained deeper and more resonant.

What had happened? Warren wondered. Clearly, some profound shift had occurred, but what, how? He had promised his parents he would spend a year working at their farm in Fresno. He used that time to study at the county hospital library. Night after night he would spend hours reading and researching.

At the end of the year he went back to L.A. and began to incorporate what he had learned. He believed he could now heal through treating the voice. Using the technique he had stumbled upon by accident—inducing a paraconscious state— he believed he could now detect energy patterns in parts of the body, brain, and nervous system, and break through old energy blockages. In so doing, he believed, new energies could be freed.

Warren explained, "I noticed that there was a microsecond of time delay between vocal effort and vocal response. Between the moment when a person marshaled inner resources to produce a sound and the moment when that sound was actually produced, there was an interruption. Something was assembling in the body to resist the vocal response. I called this phenomenon the 'collapse rate,' because when people attempted to produce the vocalization from complete openness, they could not do it. Instead, they would revert to a conditioned response from the past in which the body would actually collapse into itself. Only then could they produce the sound."

I knew I should have paid more attention in physics class; I was lost. I begged him to simplify it for me.

"This is a subtle event," Warren explains, "It happens in the blink of an eye and almost always is unconscious to the individual. To me, however, it was very apparent. At first, I didn't understand fully why it was happening, but I had clear intuition and sensitivity to such things and believed, whatever it was, that it was critical."

93

"Critical to what?"

"In order to fully engage the voice, I had to get an immediate response, not a delayed response. A delayed response would always block the full expression of the voice. So I had to get the student to produce the sound before he could revert to a conditioned response. I did this by applying pressure to certain points and at the same time, rapidly repositioning the body to change the breath pattern."

Joe left the next day. In the afternoon, Mark, another student, arrived from Seattle. Also a singer-composer, Mark was married, with two small children. Once seriously overweight and told by doctors that he was well on his way to the diabetes and heart problems that ran in his family, Mark had worked hard to lose seventy pounds.

"My first meeting with Warren, after nothing more than a hello and a handshake, he could tell me that the voice I was using was not my own. It was weak and small. He also intuited that my body had gone through some severe trauma and mentioned several specifics about the past and the current state of my health, things not apparent from the outside but that were accurate. I was impressed.

"I've had other experiences with altered states—drugs in my early years and meditation and yoga in recent years—where I felt I had left my body. But this was different. I really left. I felt a momentary pang of fear, but that subsided quickly. Then I tried to remember where I was. For a moment I thought I was in Vancouver, where I like to vacation. Then suddenly I was back in Warren's studio, fully aware of what had happened.

"When he picked up the hand-held machine that looked like a saber saw with a rubber-tipped end and began running it up and down my leg, it was pretty painful."

I realized something about Warren inspired enough trust in his students to put up with not only the pain but with what must be a degree of fear.

Mark says that Warren talks the whole time, explaining each step of the way why he is going after a particular area of the body. "He was unwavering in his determination to rid that area of the fear and painful emotions that he believed were stored there, preventing me from using the voice that is my birthright. When I felt I couldn't take anymore, Warren would just move to another area or give me a short break and begin again."

I asked Mark how he felt afterward.

"I was exhausted and covered in sweat. I had to lie down for an hour or so before I could make the drive home. But as my strength returned, I felt a sense of happiness and completion. I knew that something profound had happened to me. I was in an endorphin-high state, the way I feel after running a couple of miles, strong and powerful and able to do anything. I also felt extremely grateful to have had this experience, to have my friends and family and to just be alive."

It is tempting. When Warren says to me, "C'mon, let's check

95

you out," I hesitate, but my curiosity wins. He says he has been observing me, listening to my voice ever since I arrived.

He sits me in the chair and puts his hand on my neck and shoulder, feeling the tightness in the muscles. Then he picks up one of his tools and runs the edge of it along my shoulder. At first it feels good, then it begins to sting, like a hundred needles shooting into the muscle.

Watching my face closely, judging my reaction, he slowly increases the pressure. "Breathe," he says. Now he moves it down my arm below my elbow, and it really hurts. He stops a moment. Then he props my leg up and covers it with a towel, and using a smaller instrument that he calls a "percussion," he runs it along my tibia bone. I cry out. "Whoa! Stop!"

Warren explains that is where my energy is blocked, and that it is releasing now. He asks if I can I take a little more.

I smile bravely. "I'll try," I say. But then, he bends me forward and tells me to take a deep breath and hold it while he bends me backward.

I feel dizzy and lightheaded, as if I'm going to pass out. I'm chicken. I can't do it. Not this time, anyway. Yet that night, my dreams are rich and vivid. And the next day, my mind feels scrubbed clean.

It is my last day at Warren's. A tall, rugged man appears at the back door in jeans and boots and a cap, a bandana around his neck. A cowboy or workman, I assumed. Warren had been having some repairs on the house. The man was neither.

Rick, the husband of Warren's housekeeper, had come for a session.

Three and a half years ago, at the age of forty-eight, Rick was diagnosed with cancer of the stomach and pancreas. Doctors were able to operate but told him he would not survive beyond two years. Two years later, the cancer came roaring back. Rick grew up in Texas and sounds very much like a cowboy. He is eager to talk about what happened to him. "Tumors on my pancreas, liver, colon, and everywhere in between. Nine months of chemo, and I kept getting sicker and sicker. Many times I just wanted to give up."

Rick's wife insisted he come to see Warren. They had three children together; Rick had his own successful concrete business. He had everything to live for. "My wife wasn't going to let me die," he says. "She doesn't want to have to train someone else, not after all these years."

Warren suggested a nutritionist who put him on a program of herbs, vitamins, and chelation therapy to remove metals in his body. His wife juiced vegetables for him every day, made sure he took his vitamins. Then Warren got to work on him, several sessions a week, as much as Rick could handle.

Three months later, blood tests, CT scans, MRIs showed no signs of cancer. "I'm on borrowed time. I was supposed to be dead three months ago."

I ask Rick why he thinks he's beating the disease. He ponders that a moment. "Maybe it's Warren's treatments, maybe it's all     97 the alternative stuff I've been doing. Or maybe it's the damn chemo. Who knows? If I had to choose which one of the three to give up, I wouldn't know. Would you?"

As of this writing, a little more than a year later, Rick is still cancer-free.

I have asked several scientists about potential explanations for Warren's work. Psychologist David Wood used the metaphor of a computer that freezes. It has to be rebooted. "That's what Warren is doing."

Another, Robert Houston, a former engineer who played a prominent role in the design of the flight simulators used to train commercial and military pilots and who has known Warren since 1962, says, "He re-maps the brain, like the young girl and her father in the movie *Fly Away* did with the geese. He trained them to follow an airplane south. I think Warren's doing the most radical work in the field. The man's a genius."

I leave Warren's with a basket of fresh eggs and a promise to myself to work up the courage to experience those ten seconds of heaven that Joe and Mark and Rick described.

I slip my favorite Ella Fitzgerald tape into the tape deck and start to sing along. Who knows? Maybe Warren can even get me singing on pitch.

When I told Warren I couldn't sing, he said "Impossible, everyone can sing. Your voice is just stuck in the wrong side of your brain. Like Meat Loaf's when he sustained a knee injury. The trauma shut down his voice.

"In your case, the feelings you repressed as a child, and again when you were faced with a life-threatening illness, took your voice down."

As I drove, I could still feel soreness along my shinbone where Warren said the timeline was. If I really allowed him to release that blocked energy, according to Warren, I would find my real voice.

When I got home, I called to thank him and to make an appointment for sessions before the end of the year. Maybe in time to go caroling.

# CHAPTER
# TEN

# "BUNDJI"

## GERRY BOSTOCK

Did I ever tell you how I found the other half of my bear?" It was Howard Wills on the phone. "Your *what?*" Sometimes because of his southern drawl I misunderstand an occasional word. I could have sworn he said "bear."

"My bear stone. In 1998 up at Black Mountain in North Carolina, I was giving a meditation and healing retreat for the Cherokees, and I met an Aboriginal healer."

It seems that one of the local women approached Howard and invited him to her house for dinner. She said she wanted him to meet another healer from Australia who had come to work with the Cherokee children.

That night they stood talking in the kitchen—the woman,

the Australian, and Howard. Howard had forgotten he had his hand in his pocket. He was fiddling loose change and felt a small stone. He took it out of his pocket and looked at it. He remembered the stone, a green fluorite in the shape of a bear that he had found many months before at Mount Shasta in California.

The Australian looked at it, a strange expression crossed his face, and he reached into his shirt and pulled out a deerskin medicine bag, a gift from the Cherokees. He reached inside the bag and extracted a stone, also a green fluorite, and also broken. The two healers looked at them, amazed, and realized the two pieces fit and together formed a perfect bear.

"Brother!" they called out in unison, and hugged.

They have stayed in touch ever since. Howard urged me to call Gerry in Sydney to find out when he might be in the States again so I could meet him. From time to time over the next few months I would try the number Howard gave me. It didn't work. Frustrated, I was unable to contact him.

Then one day I called a friend who lived on the Gold Coast and asked if she had a Sydney phonebook. She found another number. This time I got Gerry's nephew, who said Gerry was somewhere in the States, but he almost never called in for messages. I left one anyway.

A day later, the phone rang. A husky voice with an unmistakable Australian accent asked for me. It was Gerry Bostock. Polite, a bit shy, he explained he was in Oakland, California. I told him Howard's story about the bear stone, and he laughed and said, "Yes, it's true. I always knew I had a brother somewhere there in the States."

In his sixties, Gerry is smallish, five-seven, and round. He is all in sepia, except for the eyes, which are dark and penetrating and seem to reach deep into the soul of whoever he is talking to. Over the next few weeks I learned his story.

Gerry Bostock is his English name; he has tribal names too, but his close friends call him "Bundji." He was born in Grafton, New South Wales, in 1942. His mother is a Bundjalung from the Nymboida Aboriginal Reserve. His father is a Mulunjali tribesman from southeastern Queensland, a part of the Bundjalung Nation.

Most of his father's generation lived on church missions and government reserves, much like the Indian Reservations in North America in the 18th and 19th centuries. Like the Native Americans, Aboriginals were subjected to the whims of the state and church. Undereducated, the men became cheap farm labor; the women domestic servants. At the time, state officials could take Aboriginal children away at any time, with or without their parents' consent. "White Australians," he explained, "commonly referred to this as 'Nigger Farming.'

"Children were sent to government-sponsored labor training schools; younger ones were taken to orphanages and adopted by white Australian families."

Gerry's father, refusing to raise his family under those condi-    103 tions, moved away, finding work wherever he could. Gerry, meanwhile, stayed with his father's parents at Tweed Heads, on the far north Australian coast.

His grandparents taught Gerry about spirituality and healing. One uncle was a gifted clairvoyant, another uncle used to "throw the bones." "He had a small bag containing an assortment of bones," Gerry explained, "that he would shake and then cast on the floor to forecast future events. Whether they were human bones or not, no one would say, but I was always taken from the room when he used them. Perhaps for my own safety, in case any malevolent spirits came through."

Tribal elders—Cleverfellers, the Aboriginal name for shamans— visited his grandfather regularly. One of Gerry's earliest memories is being brought with other children before a dying elder who would choose which child he would be responsible for in the spirit world. That child would be looked after and protected his whole life. Then, when that child died, the guardian would reincarnate.

Gerry's teachings and training by healers began when he was four years old, but they told him he would forget much of what they had taught him until the day when he was ready.

He finished school, spent nine years in the Army, and became a political activist. He was among the first Aboriginal delegation to visit the People's Republic of China in 1972.

Gerry is a natural storyteller. In our conversations he spoke vividly and with wonderful, whimsical humor. I was not surprised when he told me about his brief, but apparently successful, career as a writer.

He wrote poetry and plays first, becoming one of the founding members of the Black Theatre in Sydney. Then he turned his talents to filmmaking, producing and directing a documentary, *Lousy Little Sixpence*. In 1984, he flew to the Soviet Union to the Tashkent Film Festival to accept an award for the documentary.

But that was not to be his life. Something happened to him that Gerry took to be a lesson from Spirit about his future. He had gone out into the bush to set up camp and to work on a screenplay. Sitting by the campfire, pen and notebook at hand, a "willy-nilly" (a small spiraling wind) blew up, forcing him to pack up camp and move.

He found a cave that seemed ideal and he stayed there working for nine weeks.

"One late afternoon, as I rode my bike back to the cave, I noticed a beautiful, golden glow all around me and thought it must be from an unusually beautiful sunset. But when I looked I realized the sun had already gone below the horizon. I wondered if the glow was from the moon, but the moon had not yet risen.

"I noticed the light had formed an amber arc around me. It shone as bright as a spotlight and seemed to keep pace with the speed I was traveling on my bicycle. I glanced into the bush and noticed that it had gotten quite dark. When I steered the bike to dodge potholes in the road, the light would move with me. So I looked skyward to see if it was from a police helicopter trying to spot drug crops in the bush. Nothing.

"Then I noticed the strangest thing of all: the arc of light had no beam, no apparent source. And then it struck me. The light was coming from me! My entire body was glowing with it."

He said he had a dream that night, a dream that explained what had happened to him and what the light meant.

"I was with my Aboriginal teachers once more. They asked me if I was ready to accept my true path, the path of a healer. I said I was. They asked me to recall all they had taught me many years before. The knowledge came flooding in. They then began to instruct me about how to heal with love and light, with crystals and energy. They taught me how to feel energy in the environment and how to channel that into a person needing healing.

"What stood out most of all was the heat. My hands became like the coils of a stove. In the dream my teachers showed me several people who needed healing. I placed my hands upon them and their bodies vibrated with intensity as the energy surged through them.

"When I woke in the morning I knew it was not just a dream. I believe the spirit teachers who appeared to me took me into another dimension, to a place where time and space as we know it have no meaning. For the first time I really felt my body. I knew something had changed but I was not sure how or what had changed."

"Was that when your life as a healer began?" I asked.

"Not right away," he said.

Gerry returned to Sydney first and completed the script and continued to work in film and television, but he knew he had been directed now toward his true path.

I asked him how people found out about his healing abilities.

He had no idea, he said. He certainly hadn't put out the word. People just started showing up asking for help. Gerry believes Spirit had sent them. "When I placed my hands on someone in need of healing, my hands became incredibly hot, exactly the same as in the cave dream."

Inevitably, the subject of money comes up. Stories had circulated recently about a well-known healer who had begun to charge large sums of money, and according to the story, his powers were taken away. Native American medicine people often told me that the lure of "frog skins" was a dangerous one. I asked Gerry how he felt about this complicated issue. Does becoming a healer mean living on donations? Trinkets? Pouches of tobacco?

Gerry explained that while he still worked in film and television, he had no need to charge anything, but as more and more people came to him and he began to do his healing full time, he had to be paid something. Until then, there had always been an exchange: an artist would give Gerry a piece of artwork, a writer might create a poem. All cultures have some traditional form of exchange. As Gerry saw it, money was just another form of energy.

People who know Gerry say he never asks for a specific sum. He accepts whatever is offered. Interestingly, according to his friends, people with the most money offer less than those with little. I would hear this again during my travels. Healing has to do with spirituality, after all. Is there some sort of biblical conclusion to be drawn from this?

Gerry began to attend workshops and healing conferences, meeting healers of other indigenous cultures—Native American, African, Filipino, Maori. They would sit all night together exchanging ideas and teachings. One day, Gerry took a group on a day trip out to the bush about thirty miles from Sydney, to what used to be an old Aboriginal village. As they approached, they could hear singing and talking from the campsite and the sounds of children playing. But when they got there, it was completely empty.

In May 1996, Gerry made his first trip to the States. He stayed a year, traveling across the country, meeting with medicine people of various tribes and non-Native healers as well. He found there were many people in need of healing but not enough traditional healers to help them. When he returned to Australia, people e-mailed and called begging him to return to the States. He would eventually, but not for two more years. Instead he did distance healings on the telephone, which, according to reports, seemed almost as effective as his in-person work.

Gerry and I discovered our paths had crossed before. In 1991, when I had received my breast cancer diagnosis, Bear Heart, a Navajo medicine man whom I had interviewed for a previous book, insisted on coming into the operating room with me for the biopsy procedure. One of my doctors agreed; the other, one I would have sworn was a Native American, rolled his eyes and muttered something about chicken feathers.

Right about that time, Gerry was traveling through New Mexico. Someone took him to meet Bear Heart. "It was in a restaurant in Old Albuquerque," Gerry recalled, "just outside a reservation. We talked for a while and then he asked me to do a healing on him. He said his legs and his back had been giving him a great deal of discomfort. So I worked on him in the car parked outside the restaurant. I had the feeling he was just checking me out."

After that, Bear Heart invited Gerry to go with him to the Navajo reservation outside of Gallup, a five-hour drive from Albuquerque, to assist in the healing of a boy with brain damage.

The ceremony, held in a hogan (a six-sided building), lasted from sundown to sunrise the next morning. "Fifteen to twenty Navajos were there, seated in a circle, singing and praying. Each person would take a pinch of ground peyote on their tongue and sip some tea, also made from peyote. Grandfather Bear

Heart did a traditional blessing on the boy. Then he invited Gerry to do his healing. By morning, the boy was showing marked improvement.

"Before leaving, Ruby, Grandfather Bear Heart's sister, gave a very emotional speech," Gerry said. "She thanked me for the healing I did on her son and said that it had made us brothers. In front of all those gathered she declared me her adopted son. Grandfather presented me with a Navajo healing blanket and an eagle feather."

Word that I was writing about Gerry's work somehow got on the "moccasin telegraph," and before long my e-mail box was full of letters from people all over the country who had been healed by Gerry—people with broken limbs or broken hearts, lives so shattered that sometimes Gerry would weep: a woman with epilepsy who had been having thirty seizures a day; a diabetic whose legs had turned black and was told he had to have them amputated. I called and spoke with several of them. I kept in touch with some over a period of months and tracked their progress. Their stories were heartfelt and persuasive.

I kept hearing about something Gerry does that people refer to as the "Bundjalung Tickle." A misnomer, apparently, since I'm told it is quite painful. I asked Gerry what it was. He laughed and said, "Oh they're telling on me, are they? It's what I do to send energy down through the body starting at the upper clavicle. I guess it is a bit painful for a second, like a bolt of lightning that lasts maybe five seconds, or until the energy is released."

I asked where he learned that particular technique.

"From the Mob. They taught me everything."

"The mob? What mob?"

"The Bundjalung Mob. You know, the Tribe upstairs."

Gerry spent a month in Cordova, a fishing village in Southeast Alaska, where people were still suffering from the effects of the Exxon *Valdez* disaster some years before. Cordova holds the dubious distinction of appearing in *The Guinness World Book of Records* for having the highest concentration of alcoholism in its population.

He met an artist there, Jen-Ann Krechmeier, who had heard from a Native elder of the Eyak tribe that a great Aboriginal healer was coming to Anchorage. Jen-Ann, who had lived with pain all her life, had spent much of her childhood in a body cast and a wheelchair. She always believed that in her forty-ninth year an Aboriginal healer would drop down out of the sky and take away her pain. She didn't know if that information had come to her in a dream or if she just knew it, but the phone call from an Eyak elder came just months away from her fiftieth birthday.

Jen-Ann flew from her home in Cordova to Anchorage in the middle of a blizzard and went to the elder's home to meet the healer.

"Gerry seemed to float into the room," Jen-Ann remembers. "I looked into his eyes and felt this was the healer I had an appointment with all my life."

111

They sat around a table and talked for a while, then Gerry reached over and put his hand on her right side, the damaged side, and told her he could feel an energy leak.

When Jen-Ann got up on the massage table, Gerry told her the spirit of an aborted child—a boy—was still in her and told her how to meet his spirit and send it into the light. He also saw the alcohol and drugs she began using at thirteen to blank out the pain of her mother's death and her subsequent alienation from the rest of her family.

His powerful hands worked deep into tissue and joints, at times so painfully Jen-Ann had to cry out. Gerry explained he would go as deep as she was willing. "Everyone has the right to hang onto their 'stuff,' but if you want it gone, it'll be gone!"

Gerry's belief, from the teachings he received "from the Mob," is that all illness, all disorders, are connected to our relatives—a brother, sister, parents, grandparents. He is able to see that connection while he is working and often stuns the person he is working on with accurate information about a relative or ancestor.

As he worked on Jen-Ann, she felt a peace enter her body, and the burden of her life felt as if it had been lifted from her. She could forgive her parents, the men who had abused her. She saw light streaming from them and "all at once I realized how incredibly loved we are by God, that we block ourselves off from this love with our old anger, resentment, and petty judgments."

Gerry worked on her for two-and-a-half hours, then asked her to stand. The pain was gone. All of it. After the treatment, Jen-Ann and a friend went to a shopping mall. "I could run! For the first time in so many years, I could run!"

That was in 1988. She is still free of pain, physical and emotional. They have spoken on the phone many times. Sometimes he counsels her and when needed, he does a distance healing.

Jen-Ann says, "It's about love."

# CHAPTER
## ELEVEN

# CHIROPRACTOR
## TO THE STARS

### RUTH ZIEMBA

Like many people, my back occasionally gets out of align-
ment. Sometimes badly; other times with just a twinge or a
dull ache. I ignore it if I can. If it gets worse, though, I go to a
chiropractor, get adjusted, and it's better. Until the next time.

At lunch one day with Dom and Carol DeLuise, the conversation got around to backs and Dom started talking about
Dr. Ruth. Not the sex one; this Dr. Ruth is a chiropractor,
but she practices a totally different kind of chiropractic. "She's
a genius with backs," Dom said. I took the card and filed it
away.

One day soon after, I leaned down to pick up Tashi, my five-
pound puppy, and couldn't get up.

Creeping Quasimodo-like across the room to my desk, I rifled through the drawer to find the card. I called. The back gods were smiling on me. Dr. Ruth had a cancellation; she could see me that day.

"The other Dr. Ruth" is a petite 44-year-old who looks like a teenager. Her office sits at the top of a hill in the Pacific Palisades, near Santa Monica. The building is rustic and casual, with each office opening onto a deck that overlooks the Santa Monica Mountains. Before we begin, Dr. Ruth and I sit at one of the tables on the deck and talk. Her small dog, a Jack Russell named Angel who comes with her to the office, plays at our feet.

Dr. Ruth is soft-spoken and polite. She asks about my medical history and I ask her to explain what she does, but I am in too much pain to hear it all. Something about nerve pathways and fluid flow and mountain streams, which all sound wonderful. Let it begin.

We go inside to her front office where a young assistant sits at a computer scheduling appointments. Just behind the assistant is a room with three leather massage tables. The one by the window is empty. Shoes are left at the door, but I am fully clothed as Dr. Ruth asks me to lie face down on the table, relax and breathe, while she spends a minute or two with the person on the table next to me. I lie there listening to the soft music and watching Angel watch me.

Dr. Ruth comes back. First she touches a spot on the back of my neck, quickly, with gentle pressure, then moves to another spot on my tailbone. Both spots are far removed from my pain. Angel, the Jack Russell, rolls onto her back hoping for a tummy rub. "I would if I could," I whisper.

The people occupying the other tables are face up, their hands folded over their forehead or over their abdomen. I wonder what they are doing.

A moment later, Dr. Ruth asks me to turn over, lie face up. She places my hands, one on top of the other, on my forehead and tells me to take three breaths. In the nose, out the mouth. She then places my hands on my sternum, then over my navel, breathing in and out three times at each spot.

This is part of the Twelve Stages of Healing, Dr. Ruth explains. This practice brings heightened awareness to areas that are disconnected. "This is how we find the leaks."

*Leaks?*

"Places where energy seeps out. Think of it as the windshield wipers of your life, clearing away the years of accumulated dirt that have been clouding your vision into every area of your life. Once cleared, your ability to focus will increase and so will your energy level. Your coping mechanisms will improve and so will your relationships. Your backaches will ease and so will your headaches. Your future will be more about responding fully to life instead of defending yourself against it."

My eyes are closed.

I feel heat on my stomach. I wonder if she is using a heat     117 lamp. I open my eyes. She is not holding anything; the heat is coming from her hands, which she holds at least two feet above me.

She asks me to sit up. Centering my head so that it sits erect and straight on my shoulders, Dr. Ruth runs her hands down my spine, puts one finger on my neck again, and says, "That's better." I stand up and bend forward, turning slightly right and to the left. Smiling, she asks, "How do you feel?"

I tell her the pain is gone, but I wonder to myself if it will come back as soon as I leave the office. It doesn't. Not that night, not the next morning.

I have explained to Dr. Ruth that I am a journalist and that I would like to learn more about this odd brand of chiropractic practice.

"Anytime," she says, and gives me a parting hug.

Several days later my back is still better. Unlike other chiropractors I had been to, there was no bone cracking. I had to know—what did she do?

The following week—still pain-free—I sit with her on her deck sipping tea. I ask her how she came upon this technique.

Ruth Ziemba was born and raised in a small town on the outskirts of Springfield, Mass. She earned her bachelor's degree in nursing at the University of Utah, then began her career as an oncology nurse at the Dana Farber Cancer Institute in Boston. She became a staff member at the Body/Mind Research Group at Boston's Beth Israel Hospital, which was led by Joan Borysenko. It was there that she began to see illness in a new way. She wanted to know more about the mind-body connection.

Later that year Ruth had a car accident that left her with severe back pain. She saw a chiropractor and after a few sessions decided she would like to learn more. After careful investigation of various systems of chiropractic—she didn't like the sound of bones cracking—she found one called Network Spinal Analysis, developed twenty years before by Dr. Donald Epstein in New York. For the next few years, Ruth shared an office in Beverly Hills with Epstein's main instructor, Dr. Michael Stern. Under his tutelage, Ruth learned to integrate the use of the breath into her practice.

"What was his system? Did he do adjustments?" I ask.

"Yes, but his adjustments were subtle and precise. Just a touch and release at a point on the sacrum, and slight, quick pressure on the neck and along the spine. What these adjustments do is to connect the body's rhythms through breath, touch, and movement. When the tension melts, the shoulders give way, and one has a sense of fluidity, clarity."

"But how can such slight pressure release tension?" I ask.

"Because it directly affects the nervous system—the brain and the spinal cord. The barest touch to the upper neck . . ." She reaches over and touches the base of my skull, "may be all it takes to release tension in the lower spine. When tension is released from the nervous system, it's released from your entire body."

119

I press her to be more specific. "Is the whole nervous system located in the spine?"

"Your spine shows where you are holding on to psychological and physical trauma in your life. The musculature takes on a character of thickness that's associated with the length of time since the trauma occurred. So your spine develops a barrier, a protective wall."

Dr. Ruth stands behind me and demonstrates. "I can feel along the backbone and see exactly where the trauma lives, how long ago it happened, and at what age."

That sounded quite amazing. "You can? Really?" I ask. "And can a person feel when trauma is settling into the backbone?"

"How many time have you found yourself in a stressful situation and said, 'I'll just push it to the back of my mind. I'll deal with the tension later'?"

"Many times. Probably more than I know."

"Well, what *is* the back of your mind? It's your spine, your nervous system. It's where tension is stored. The body remembers."

"And that tension creates back pain?"

"That tension creates all kinds of pain. When we are under any kind of stress—emotional, physical, or mental—our brain is going to make a decision: Do I need to amplify this impulse to feel? Or do I need to annihilate it? For instance, when a person goes into shock, it's because the information is too much for the body, so the body shuts itself down."

"And what does that look like to you?" I ask.

"Have you ever seen someone walking with their shoulders all rounded looking like they're in a lot of pain? If you ask them, they may say they feel fine. Well, actually that is because they are not feeling that area of their body at all. It's not safe to. That's how our system protects us."

"So do you then have to break through that protective shield?"

"There is a connective tissue that covers our brain and spinal cord, and that tissue, along with the muscle tissue, stores memories. When this tissue tightens, our spine, which has the ability to stretch, is restricted."

"And just those quick, light touches are all it takes to break through?" My session with her had lasted all of about fifteen minutes.

"There are some highly responsive people who just by holding their hand can trigger a release. What we're talking about is creating a global effect in the body. There are areas that store tension in the body and other areas that are freer. Areas that are freer can actually assist the areas that aren't as free.

"But, in order to fix something we must first be able to find it. As our brain is better able to inventory the body, it can better orchestrate healing. This occurs naturally as we become more aware of our spinal tension patterns. Those who have had the greatest wounds and traumas and have stored tension or blocked energy can develop new strategies to access healing. This is part of the "stress busting" effect demonstrated in Spinal Network

121

Care. Actually, the greater the wound, the greater the potential gift."

She tells me about a woman who came to her with such bad TMJ (temporo-mandibular joint syndrome, a clenching of the jaw) that she couldn't even eat a sandwich. After one session her face physically changed.

"And did it stay changed?" I ask.

"What I have observed is that when tension is released it stays released. New stresses come into our lives, of course; it's how we handle them that changes."

Just then, a couple I recognize from a TV sitcom comes walking onto the deck holding an infant that looks to be fresh out of the oven. Jokingly, I ask if the baby has come for an adjustment. "Yes," Dr. Ruth answers, "It was a traumatic birth and the baby is colicky."

"She wakes up every hour," the mother says. "We're exhausted."

I ask Dr. Ruth what she can do with a newborn and she invites me to come into the office to watch.

The woman lies on the table with the infant face down on her stomach. Dr. Ruth performs the same quick light touches on the baby she did on me. Then she holds her hands a foot or so above mother and child for a moment. The baby gurgles.

The system Dr. Ruth uses seems to work. But the secret ingredient, the one she hadn't explained, is Dr. Ruth herself and those heat-lamp hands of hers. I have not had any back problems for many months, and I've noticed when I walk Tashi, my stride seems a bit freer, my back a little straighter. And when I become stressed, I try to remember not to let tension settle in my spine. But if it ever does and I feel the familiar tightening of the neck and shoulders, I think about Dr. Ruth and those quick, light touches, and I breathe.

I did not know that I would be putting it all to the test so quickly. A call soon came from my mother's caregiver in Palm Beach at 5:00 A.M. Sometime during the night, my mother had passed away. I call Bill, the only one of my sons who lives in L.A. and who volunteered to be the one to go with me, and he picks me up on the way to the airport later that morning.

# CHAPTER
## TWELVE

# THE PLACEBO EFFECT:

## THE LIE

## THAT HEALS

Death had stalked my mother for more than two years. Stalked and teased her, hiding behind the door, then poking his head out now and then to remind her she was not, as she liked to say, invincible. Death had to tiptoe to her bedside and grab her while she slept. And I was not there to say good-bye.

When my father died, twenty-five years earlier, I was devastated, my grief bottomless. Now, on the plane with my son on the way to Florida, I felt numb. We had not had an easy time of it, my mother and I, and no matter how hard we tried to mend the torn fabric of our relationship, we never could. The fabric could never be mended now.

125

It rained the night we arrived, a hard, angry rain. We met my cousin and her son for dinner. As we left the restaurant, I slipped on the rain-slicked pavement and fell forward, my face striking the ground. Blood gushed from my nose.

In exactly the way Dr. Ruth had explained to me only a week earlier, I set aside my feelings to deal with them at some later date. And just as she said, the trauma went straight to my spine. My back went out.

The funeral, the blur of faces, lawyers.

All the magic I had been collecting over the past year vanished. I had crossed back into the realm of what my mother called the "real world."

Maybe the magic was only a placebo.

Often during my research on healing I had wondered, How much of what I am seeing is the placebo effect in action? And is there an element of the placebo effect in all medicine?

Described by Harvard University scientist Dr. Anne Harrington as "the lie that heals," the word placebo is Latin for "I shall please." A placebo looks like an active drug, but has no pharmacological properties of its own. Yet, mysteriously, when given under the right conditions or by the right doctor—or healer—a placebo can affect healing.

One well-reported case of the placebo effect dates back to 1957. A "Mr. Wright" was hospitalized in Long Beach, California, suffering through the final stages of lymphatic cancer. X-rays showed large tumors the size of baseballs in his chest and abdomen. Almost a liter of fluid had to be drawn from his chest every day. Doctors considered him untreatable. But Wright, who made a daily practice of reading medical journals, learned that his doctor's clinic had been chosen to evaluate a horse serum called Krebiozen that had been thought to be effective against cancer. Because of the advanced stage of his cancer, Wright was not considered eligible for the program. Still, he begged his primary physician, Dr. Philip West, to give him the drug.

Finally, figuring there was nothing to lose, his doctor relented and gave Wright his first injection on a Friday. The following Monday, Wright was up and around, laughing and joking with the nurses. Of all his test subjects, Dr. West found that only Wright had shown improvement. "Wright's tumor masses had melted like snowballs on a hot stove." Within ten days of the first treatment, Wright was discharged from his "deathbed."

Wright continued to follow the evaluation, in medical journals and newspapers, of the "miracle" drug that had saved his life. But about a month later, new findings reported that Krebiozen had been shown to be ineffective. Almost immediately Wright had a relapse and the tumors returned.

Dr. West decided to play a hunch. He told Wright that the newspapers were mistaken about Krebiozen and that a new, super-refined, double-strength supply was due to arrive the following day. Wright was ecstatic. The doctor delayed treatment with the "new" batch until he felt Wright's anticipation had reached a peak. The doctor then gave Wright an injection of *water*.

Following the placebo injection, Wright's second recovery proved even more dramatic than the first. Once again, the tu-

127

mors melted, his chest fluid vanished, and he resumed a normal life. Over the next two months Dr. West continued the injections of plain, ordinary water, and Mr. Wright remained symptom-free—until he read a conclusive report published by the AMA declaring that Krebiozen was totally worthless in the treatment of cancer. Two days later, Mr. Wright died.

Once dismissing it as quackery, modern science is discovering the power of the placebo effect. Using the latest techniques of brain imagery, doctors can watch how a thought, a belief, and expectation of a cure can actually cause a change. Similarly, in experiments around the world, smelling a placebo helped asthmatic children in Venezuela increase their lung function by thirty-three percent. In Japan, people exposed to fake poison ivy developed real rashes. In 1994, at the Houston Veteran's Medical Center in Texas, a surgeon, Dr. J. Bruce Moseley, performed ten sham arthroscopic knee surgeries in which he made an incision in the knee but did nothing. Two years later, patients who underwent the sham surgery reported the same relief of pain and swelling as those who had the real surgery.

In a series of studies reported in *New York Times Magazine* ("The Placebo Prescription," January 9, 2000), doctors successfully eliminated warts by painting them with a brightly colored, inert dye and promising patients the warts would be gone when the color wore off. In another study of asthmatics, researchers found that they could produce dilation of the airways by simply telling people they were inhaling a bronchiodilator, even when they weren't.

The placebo effect also works in reverse. The term for that is *nocebo*. In a 1983 study, one control group was given chemotherapy drugs while another group was given sugar pills. Thirty percent of the group who were given sugar pills lost their hair. The placebo effect was powerful enough to cause hair loss in patients who simply *believed* that they had taken a chemotherapy drug.

What are we seeing here? Is modern science just beginning to catch onto the principles that have been in use by indigenous healers throughout the world for centuries? I was about to find out. My next quest involved the phenomena of "sleight-of-hand" surgery in the Philippines and "psychic surgery" in Brazil. I couldn't wait to get back to the world of magic.

# CHAPTER

## THIRTEEN

# BEYOND

# PLACEBO

## HENRY BELK

I had been hearing the name Henry Belk almost from the time I began my research on healers. William Henry Belk, Jr.'s father was the founder of the Belk's Department Store chain in the South, and Henry, following his graduation from Duke University, had dutifully taken the reins. But when his teenage daughter drowned in a tragic accident, Henry began a lifelong quest. He created the Belk Foundation for Psychical Research and turned his house into a treasury of information on psychics and healing.

I called him one day, told him about my project, and asked a question or two. I don't remember what one question was exactly, but I do remember his answer: "If you're really interested, get on a plane and come down. You can't learn anything in a phone call." He gave me his address and told me I could come anytime. "But it better be soon, I don't plan to be around much longer."

A week later, I flew to Durham, North Carolina, and rang Henry's doorbell. Eighty-four and painfully thin, his mane of white hair uncombed, he greeted me as if he knew me. Henry lived alone—well, not quite alone. A huge cat darted through the room and flew down the stairs to the basement as I arrived. The room I entered was surrounded by floor-to-ceiling stacks of books and file cabinets. With a razor-sharp mind and astounding memory, Henry wasted no time.

We would begin each morning poring over text, examining photographs, some of which were yellowed and cracked with age. Hour after hour he would stand over his Xerox machine insisting that I have copies of just about everything. "I've been accumulating this stuff for over six decades; someone better make use of it."

Evenings were spent watching video footage, first of psychic surgeons in the Philippines, then in Brazil. From time to time he would reach for the phone—no matter what the hour—to call his friend Harvey Martin, author of *The Secret Teachings of the Espiritistas*. Harvey had lived for six years in the Philippines and came to know several healers, among them the psychic surgeon Alex Orbito.

The images on the videos were surprisingly sharp. In one, a

man with a serious shoulder injury that would not heal is lying on a makeshift operating table in the small back room of a nondescript clinic outside Manila. There are no scalpels, no forceps, no clamps or separators, and no suturing instruments. Alex Orbito enters the room and begins. Using only his bare hands, he begins to knead the man's shoulder until there is a sudden "popping" sound.

Then, Alex's fingertips appear to penetrate the skin. The camera zooms in closer to reveal only a few drops of blood. Then, folding back both the skin and muscles to expose the joint, we see Alex reach in and pull a piece of tissue from the shoulder socket.

I have turned away. But Henry insists I watch Alex press the opened skin back together and wipe away the last traces of blood with a cloth. A close-up shows no scar or sign of entry. The operation had lasted only three minutes; the patient said he felt no pain. Alex shows the man a piece of bloody tissue about the size of a fingertip. He explains that scar tissue had formed when the shoulder was first dislocated, preventing the joint from reconnecting properly.

The narrator of the video explains that Reverend Alex Orbito is a third-generation Philippine psychic healer and has been healing people since the age of fourteen. His grandparents founded the church where Alex sometimes works.

Henry says to me, "Of course doctors in the States believe psychic surgery is voodoo and think that Americans who go

133

there should have their heads examined. They'd like to see these healers thrown in prison for medical malpractice."

Psychic surgery dates back to the 1600s, to the *Spiritist* movement that existed in the Philippines long before the Spanish brought Christianity to its shores. According to this tradition, spirits of surgeons who lived before incorporate the body of a healer while he or she is in trance. The healer does not typically even remember performing the surgery. Once out of trance, the healer returns to his normal life.

Early Spanish settlers, viewing the practice as a form of witchcraft, routinely tortured and killed shamans and burned all *Spiritist* ritual material.

Eventually Filipinos found a way to blend their shamanism with Christianity and determined that the spirit who worked through the friars was the same God they called *Bathala*. Their healing practices, using mediums to channel doctors from the spirit world, were performed openly and have since become a part of their tourist economy. According to Harvey Martin, today there are more than a hundred thousand healers in the Philippines, many of them wealthy.

The video's narrator told of case after case of medically documented cures of diseases ranging from hay fever to cancer. What I found interesting was that early researchers into the enigma of psychic surgery found a parallel between the healing that often actually occurred and a medical mystery now known as the placebo effect.

In his book, Harvey Martin writes about an incident told to him by Alex Orbito. Harvey had taken notice of the gold Rolex Alex was wearing and asked about it.

It seems that the king of Saudi Arabia had flown Alex to his palace in order to try to heal his brother, who had a serious intestinal disorder. Alex was the last resort. In a private meeting, the king told Alex that he would reward him with a large sum of money and other gifts if he could cure his brother. Then he warned Alex that if his brother died while under his care, Alex would be beheaded.

Alex retired to his guest quarters in the palace to pray and to meditate. After several hours Alex made his decision and announced he was ready to help the king's brother. Alex was brought to the room where he performed psychic surgery on different areas of the king's brother's body. When he finished, Alex was led back to his quarters. After what seemed an eternity, Alex heard a knock on his door. Two armed guards silently escorted him to the king. Alex began to worry until he saw the smiling face of the king. The king told him that he had done well and gave Alex a large sum of money and a Rolex watch with an Arabian coat of arms emblazoned on the face. The money was used to build a healing center in Quezon City.

"Before the actual healing, I feel a certain coldness in my forehead, which gradually spreads to my whole body . . . Then, a surge of heat gravitates into my palms to signal my readiness for the operation," says Alex.

135

"When I put my hand inside the body, my hand is like a magnet. So, even if the sickness is a distance from my hand, it is drawn to me and I feel a current. When I feel the current, I know that the sickness is now in my hand and I remove it immediately. That is why the operations don't last very long. It is not I who opens the body, but the Spirit. The power emanates from God and is channeled through my hands."

Was all this psychic surgery I was watching sleight of hand? Sleight-of-hand surgery is common in the Phillipines and elsewhere. Here, the healer creates the illusion of removing a tumor. To do this he uses cleverly concealed animal blood and tissue, usually small pieces of chicken liver or gizzard purchased at the corner stall, and proceeds to imitate a real surgery.

"But if psychic surgery works," I ask Henry, "why would the healers use trickery?"

"Actually," Henry said, "among the early Filipinos, sleight of hand existed for centuries. The belief was that if you extract a *symbolic* object from a sick patient, the disease would disappear. The shaman never considered what he did to be deceitful. His only interest was that the patient be healed. Any and all means of healing came from Spirit, and therefore was miraculous."

"So then anyway you look at it, is it all placebo?" I asked.

Henry smiled enigmatically and shrugged his shoulders. But I left Durham more convinced than ever that *all* healing, including modern medicine, contained an element of the placebo effect. If belief and expectation is the spark that activates the immune system—whether delivered by a man in a white coat or a shaman in feathers—won't healing occur?

I had to buy an extra bag to carry the books, Xeroxed pages, and film Henry had insisted I take. His dedication and generosity moved me.

Two months later, I got a call that Henry Belk had passed away. Now he had a front row seat for his research.

# CHAPTER
## FOURTEEN

# SWIMMING WITH
# THE BUDDHA

## PETER MAXWEL

A half-mile from where I live and across the street from the supermarket where I shop lives a man who so resembles paintings of Christ that people stare as he walks by. He is reed-thin; his straight, dark blond hair is shoulder length, parted in the middle and curled slightly around his whiskered and stubbled face. His large, slate blue eyes gaze out with an expression that is, well, *Christlike*. I mention the sight of this man to a friend who lives nearby and shops at the same market. She knows immediately whom I am talking about. "That's Peter Maxwel," she says. "Former Australian Olympic swimming champion. He lives in one of those small houses down the street from the market. He's a healer now."

She tells me about a young girl in upstate New York, a paraplegic, on whom he performed an incredible healing. She had heard of other people he had healed, too.

From the Olympics to a bungalow in Southern California— quite a career move. I was intrigued.

Healers know about each other. Word travels in an underground network of sorts. They know who's real and who isn't. They can spot a charlatan a mile away. I call Howard Wills and ask if he knows Peter Maxwel. "Yeah," Howard drawls. "I know Peter. He's all right. I hear he's done some good things." I take that as the Howard Wills seal of approval and write down Peter's phone number (Howard has an encyclopedic phone book of healers) and call Peter to make an appointment.

His house sits on a quiet, tree-lined street, in the middle of similar, bungalow-type houses found in enclaves at the edges of Los Angeles. Incongruously ordinary, I think, as I ring the doorbell.

Peter greets me at the door. He wears a pair of khakis and a white Indian-type shirt and is barefoot. I remove my shoes and follow him up the stairs to the room where he works. That is where the ordinary ends.

At the top of the stairs is a photograph of a Peter with short hair, in swim trunks, an Olympic gold medal around his neck. Inside his room, the walls are hung with Indian tapestries and prayer rugs. Images of Christ, saints, artifacts, and relics picked up from his travels around the world—many from India—are placed on tabletops. Peter explains he studied with Swami

Kaleshwar, a young guru, at his ashram in Bangladore, in southern India.

We sit opposite each other in the softly lit room. In the background, Indian music plays on a tape deck. He tells me about his early years, his Australian accent somehow giving his stories an air of whimsy.

Born in 1961 in Perth, Australia, to an upper-middle-class family—but descended from the first fleet of British convicts who settled the island, he is quick to add—Peter would have followed in his father's footsteps and gone into politics or finance, but instead swam his way to another sort of life. After he attended private schools and competed in statewide breaststroke events, his father took him to London to train. At nineteen, Peter won a spot on the Australian Olympic Team. He won both a gold and a bronze medal in swimming at the 1980 Moscow Olympics, and he competed again in 1984 in Los Angeles, where he won two bronze medals.

Afterward, the University of Arizona offered him a scholarship. "I never really applied myself in college. I was depressed and angry in those years and didn't know why."

Five years later, he was back in Perth. A friend introduced him to an enclosed flotation tank filled with warm salt water that was used for meditation. Known as a deprivation or isolation tank, the device was made popular among spiritual seekers by the late scientist John Lily, who was known for his dolphin research and experiments with mind-expanding drugs.

Over the next eighteen months, Peter logged six hundred

141

hours in the silence of the tank, which he likened to being sealed up in a Buddhist cave. He claims to have seen his past lives and his deeply wounded present one. He felt the presence of God and God's wish that he wake up, just as others before him had woken up. And he desired to become healed so that he could in turn heal others. "I saw it all. I felt crushed, burned. All my demons came; I saw myself, my ego, and I knew that one of us would not get out of that tank alive: me or my ego.

"Finally I surrendered and melted into my Buddha mind. In the darkness of the tank, I saw a monk on the side of the road, his hand covering his face. He walked up to me and lifted his hood and I saw myself, smiling at me. The Buddha was no longer outside of me now. I had, as they say, killed the Buddha. Enlightenment comes in a moment; growth goes on forever. The time had come to leave to find my humanity."

The summer of 1987 was the time of the Harmonic Convergence, an astrological event in the Mayan calendar signaling the dawn of a global awakening—yet another new age to New Agers around the world, who gathered to meditate and pray for the healing of all relations and the sacredness of all life. A sort of spiritual Woodstock.

The two-day event turned several of Peter's like-minded friends into seekers. Peter's parents owned property forty-five minutes out of the city, with fruit trees and orchards and a pond deep enough to swim in. Peter went there to read and to meditate. Friends came for weekends; they discussed spiritual teachings of books they were reading. One friend had asthma and allergies and a dreadful fear of drowning. Peter took him into the pond, where the water came up to Peter's shoulders, and cradled his friend in his arms. At first his friend shook with fear, but after a while he grew quiet and lay peacefully in Peter's arms.

"I could feel something break open in his lungs, and suddenly he could breathe. I could feel it happening. The guy never had another asthma attack, and his fear of water had vanished."

This incident marked the first of other spontaneous healings. "I saw someone else's spine straighten as I held him in the water, and another person's hip joint go back into place. I didn't fully understand what was happening, but I knew it had to do with me and my water energy."

Soon others began to show up. Peter noticed that he could see problems in their energies and offered to try to help. "I realized then that I had abilities."

Asked how his parents reacted to his spiritual awakening, Peter said they didn't like it. They felt as if he had disconnected from the grid, that they were losing him. "My family looked at me as if I had gone insane. Because when you go through a rapid spiritual expansion, you are on the razor's edge; you could easily slip one way or the other. You could go insane. And I didn't have a teacher then, the protection of a master to show me the way. I was freelance." With a laugh, Peter said, "My parents probably would have understood if I had become an alcoholic or druggie like all the other kids of my generation. But *this*!"

Peter returned to the States, hitchhiking his way up and down the California coast to Mexico and to the Mayan ruins, then on to Europe and the Middle East. With nothing more than one pair of shoes, one pair of pants, two shirts, and an airline blanket in a shoulder bag, Peter walked barefoot through Greece, Egypt, and Israel, a pilgrimage, he said, to experience the ancient path. At the Wailing Wall in Israel, Palestinians in their stalls burst into tears at the sight of him and cried out, "Look! It's Jesus!"

I asked Peter how much of his appearance was consciously chosen to resemble images of Christ. The cut of his hair, the shape of the beard—was there a reason?

"I think our spirits choose images that will awaken others. Mine is of a Western male who gives his life to God. I could just as easily be a scrawny street beggar or a hippie bum if I put my hands out to beg. But instead I chose to put my hands out to touch, to heal.

"I had let my hair and beard grow out when I began my twenty-month pilgrimage and this is just the way it grew." He was wandering through Egypt during the time of the 1991 Iraq war, and, because the city was empty of tourists, Peter could spend all the time he wanted sitting in the temples meditating.

"I didn't know what would happen next. I didn't know if I'd ever make it back. I had surrendered my life to my quest.

"In '93 I wound up in London, where I met Angel, my future wife. She was a fashion model. I followed her first to New York, then to L.A." He laughs, remembering. "God said, 'Okay, Pete, you've traveled the world, done the barefoot thing, slept on top of pyramids; now we're going to give you the tough assignment. We're going to put you in a relationship.'

"'*Noooo!*' I said. 'Please not *that*! Millions have tried it and no one gets it right.' But I knew there were certain things in our culture I couldn't try to heal unless I was in a relationship. Angel helped me to ground the power I had developed, to find what is good and right in this culture.

"After we moved to L.A., people seemed to turn up, people with wounded souls. They just showed up at my door. I found I could connect with their sadness and their grief. I became aware that my thoughts had vibrations, which could reach into a person's soul and bring about a healing."

Reluctant at first to charge money, he supported himself working for company that sold nutritional products. Then he happened to attend a seminar given by motivational coach Breck Costin. When Breck asked Peter to talk about himself, he realized how difficult it was for him to claim his gift, to declare that he was a healer.

I asked him about the woman I had heard about in upstate New York who he had healed.

"It was in December of 2000, I was visiting a friend, an artist, who lived in an old farmhouse. I got a call from someone in L.A. about a young woman, Amy, who happened to live just minutes from where I was staying. The woman had been in a car accident eight years earlier. Three bones in her neck were broken and she was paralyzed from the shoulders down. They asked if I would see her.

"I'll never forget that day. It was incredibly cold and gray; it had been sleeting. There was this beautiful woman in her late twenties all wrapped up in sweaters and a blanket being brought out of the car and placed into her wheelchair. I went out to help get her into the house.

"Amy was shivering. She couldn't seem to get warm, even inside the house. We put her right next to the heater and still she shivered. She explained that her spinal cord injury affected her body temperature, and that even in ninety-degree heat she was cold.

"As we talked, Amy told me she'd had a premonition about an accident, and dreams about it all through her life—exactly the way it happened. She saw herself paralyzed, in a wheelchair."

I spoke to Amy on the phone after talking with Peter. I don't know what I expected, but I was surprised at how down-to-earth and plain talking she seemed. At the time of the accident, Amy was twenty-one, working for a Wall Street firm that also had offices in Greenwich, Connecticut, which is where the accident occurred.

I asked her about her premonition. Her first memory of it was at five. She remembers sitting in her kindergarten class, chin resting on her hand, daydreaming about a car accident and a wheelchair. From that time on, she saw it all again and again in her dreams. And then it happened.

"I wasn't even the one driving; I was in the passenger seat, so it wasn't a case of a self-fulfilling prophecy. There were three of us, no drinking, no drugs. We were going no more than thirty miles an hour when we hit a piece of black ice and skidded, first into a tree, and then we hit a stone wall. No one else was hurt.

"The moment of impact, I knew. *Here we go*, I thought. *This is it.*" The headrest broke off and hit her in the neck, breaking three bones. The accident had followed exactly the script that had played out in her dreams all those years.

When Amy regained consciousness, her body was attached to a frame, her head bolted to it. "From time to time they would flip me like a pancake and I would stare at the floor."

Doctors were blunt. They told her she would spend the rest of her life a "talking head."

Over the next eight years, she lived with an aide in upstate New York. Dozens of healers and psychics contacted her family, offering to heal her. Many she saw. "They were all bogus," Amy said. She was desperate. She needed someone, something to help her. "I wasn't hoping to jump up out of my wheelchair, I just needed to come unstuck. Spending my life as a talking head was one thing; living encased in a block of ice was worse."

In December 2000, when Peter was visiting his friend in up-state New York, he happened to call a friend who told him about a young woman who lived not five minutes from where he was staying. Phone numbers were exchanged and Amy called Peter. The moment she heard his voice she knew she had to meet him.

When he came out to the car to greet her, she liked him im-mediately. "He was warm and mellow, and I felt I could trust him."

147

Peter described the session: "I put my hand on her back feeling for the place where the energy was locked. On her mid-back, just below the ribs, I could feel it, a deep, cold freeze.

"I realized her emotional body had never released the shock of the accident. It wasn't just the spinal injury; it was fear trapped there in her body that caused her to feel cold. The girl was still in shock.

"After about fifteen minutes, Amy suddenly became fearful and anxious. She panicked. I asked her what was happening. She didn't know. But I did. I saw flashes of early traumas, way before the accident."

Amy couldn't believe it. "He knew things I had never told anyone, not even my best friend. A pregnancy when I was seventeen, animals killed in front of my house that were run over by cars. Horses I grew up around—my father was a horse breeder—my parents' divorce. I couldn't believe it.

"I could feel him pulling stuff out of my abdomen," Amy said, "and replacing it with good energy. Then he held a red glass heart against my heart."

Peter said, "Suddenly I could see waves of fear leaving her body. Fear that was keeping her from healing." The session lasted about an hour. When her aide came to pick her up, Amy felt disoriented.

Two days later, to her amazement, she began to feel warm. A week later, during her regular physical therapy session, her right shoulder unfroze and there was some movement. "Most of all, I could get through the rest of the winter without suffering the terrible pain of the cold."

Amy has physical therapy every day. Her recovery has speeded up. Her hip flexor and pelvis has movement now, and she is starting to take steps. "It's slow," she says. "It's like staring into the mirror and trying to watch your hair grow.

"I realize now I was tied to that wheelchair, actual or not. Peter helped me see life is okay. He opened my heart and made me warm again."

She is writing now, she wants to share her story with others tied to the same chair.

Peter explained that he felt he had been given keys while on his twenty-month pilgrimage to unlock some—not all—of people's blocked or frozen energies. "Some I just don't have the keys for, and I have no access to their programming. But other times I'm like a safecracker, my mind is a wheel, spinning, tumbling the mechanism to find the combination that will open the pathways."

# CHAPTER
## FIFTEEN

# BRAZIL:

# DOWN THE

# RABBIT HOLE

Among the books and papers I brought back from Durham was a video with a note taped to it with the words "WATCH THIS FIRST" in Henry's scrawl.

It was a ninety-minute documentary made by filmmaker David Sonnenschein called *Dr. Fritz: Healing the Body and Spirit.* Two photographs on the box showed a young Brazilian man and the face of an older bearded man floating beside him. The film opens on a dilapidated warehouse, with peeling paint and broken, dirty windows, in an industrial area of Rio de Janeiro. The building functions as a makeshift hospital. Hordes of people, many of whom look poor and destitute, gather inside the gates, waiting to be healed.

The camera pans the crowd: People in wheelchairs or on crutches; mothers holding their babies; a man with a growth protruding from his neck; another with a withered limb. They are waiting to see Rubens Faria, a forty-three-year-old medium who channels the spirit of Dr. Fritz, a German surgeon who died in 1915.

According to the narrator, the actual Dr. Fritz was born in Munich, Germany and became a military doctor in World War I. He died while operating on the field of battle in Estonia, when a grenade exploded.

Rubens Faria is the most recent of a string of mediums to channel Dr. Fritz. Born in São Paulo, he is a graduate of the Institute of Military Engineering, trained in computer telecommunications, and married with a young daughter.

The first person to channel Dr. Fritz's spirit was a Brazilian farmer named Arigo. In 1947, during a violent seizure, Arigo suddenly began to speak in German. Soon after, he discovered he seemed to have a knowledge of medicine and started to prescribe remedies—first for close relatives, and then for complete strangers. In 1950, he successfully performed an emergency surgery on a local politician, removing a cancerous lung tumor with only a pocket knife. News traveled quickly, and before long Arigo was treating hundreds of patients each day.

Eventually, he was charged with practicing medicine without a license and sent to prison. But soon, the sick began to line up outside the prison for treatment. In 1971, after treating the warden's daughter, Arigo was freed from prison, only to be killed in a traffic accident. A series of others channeled Dr. Fritz over the years, and each met with a sudden or violent death.

Four years later, in 1975, Dr. Fritz inhabited the body of Edvaldo Wilde, who was also killed in a traffic accident. Then, in 1980, Dr. Edson Queiroz, a gynecologist, began to channel Dr. Fritz. Three years later, he was stabbed to death in a violent argument with a former member of his staff.

I asked David Sonnenschein, the filmmaker who made the documentary on Rubens, if he had a theory about this mysterious string of violent deaths. He did not, but Rubens had told him Dr. Fritz had already warned him of his own unnatural death, which would occur four years and nine months from then (which would be December 2000).

Rubens told David he went into a terrible depression and decided he would no longer channel Dr. Fritz. He had a wife and young daughter and wanted very much to live. But then, according to Rubens, Dr. Fritz persuaded him to continue. "I am no longer afraid of death now," he told David. "When it happens, my daughter will be proud to remember that her father helped thousands of people. I will have fulfilled my mission."

(That date has come and gone and Rubens is still very much alive and continuing to channel Dr. Fritz.)

In the next scene Rubens enters a room. He is a handsome man, dressed in white, wearing thick eyeglasses. He is friendly and chats in an animated manner.

He takes his seat behind a desk and removes his glasses. Then, covering his eyes, he lets his head drop. When he looks up, his

153

face is reddish, his eyes are half-closed, and his voice is low and husky. His demeanor has changed from animated to solemn. The spirit of Dr. Adolph Fritz has apparently now entered his body.

A nurse brings him a stack of patient forms. As Dr. Fritz, Rubens has no need for the thick glasses; he rapidly sorts through the more than two hundred forms, making two piles, one for the more critical patients he will operate on first and the other for patients he will attend to later. Once finished, he heads for the operating room.

A young man sits in a wheelchair. We are told that he had been shot, rushed to a hospital, but the doctor there refused to operate. The bullet was lodged close to nerves in his neck and the surgeon feared an operation might leave him paralyzed.

Dr. Fritz begins his surgery. The young man remains seated in the wheelchair. Without anesthesia and with an unsterilized scalpel, the "doctor" makes a two-inch incision in the young man's neck. There is almost no bleeding, even as Dr. Fritz digs deeply into the young man's neck. The man is fully conscious and shows no sign of experiencing pain. Dr. Fritz cracks a joke and the young man laughs. Then, using a pair of tweezers, Dr. Fritz extracts the bullet from the patient's neck. The entire operation has taken all of five minutes.

A nurse stitches the wound and Dr. Fritz quickly moves on to a middle-aged man with a herniated disk in his back. Using the same scalpel, and again with no sterilization or anesthesia, Dr. Fritz makes a three-inch long incision near the man's lower spine. And again the patient's face shows not a trace of pain.

After that surgery, the camera follows Dr. Fritz into another room where, the narrator tells us, he will perform twenty cataract operations.

During one of the cataract surgeries, Dr. Fritz inserts a scalpel under a woman's eyelid, roughly works it back and forth while talking to the interviewer, looking only occasionally at the patient.

I fear I am going to be sick. I put the tape on pause and go splash cold water on my face.

When I return to continue viewing the tape, Dr. Fritz has finished and a nurse is putting a bandage on the woman's eye. "The woman will go home now," the narrator tells us. Apparently there is no need for recovery rooms at this hospital.

It gets worse. The narrator explains Dr. Fritz has used the same scalpel for all twenty surgeries, the same bloodied gloves, and it has taken less than thirty minutes for Dr. Fritz to perform fifteen operations.

Now a young mother is holding her baby boy, who is blind, in her arms before the camera. Dr. Fritz tells the mother to hold tight to her baby's hand. He is going to use the scalpel on *her* eyes, which are perfectly healthy.

Dr. Fritz turns and speaks in English to the camera. "This is one of the most difficult operations to perform. This is how to treat the mother for her child. I cut here, free the tissue in the mother. In two or three days, there will be no more damaged tissue in his eye. Then this baby boy can see. The mother and her baby have a very similar DNA structure, so through the

155

handholding, the change in the DNA can be transferred to the baby at the speed of light. Some children I operate on, others no, because they are too small, and I feel sorry for the baby. So I do it on the mother. Generally there is a blood tie. These chromo-somal genetic associations can transport energy. There is a chain that is electronically interlinked. You don't have to alter the whole thing, just a piece—one triggers the next and that's it."

When the operations are finished, Dr. Fritz goes to the large hall where hundreds of patients with minor complaints stand in long lines. A couple of nurses follow him, pushing a waist-high cart full of hypodermic needles. Each syringe appears to be filled with the same dark brown liquid. Dr. Fritz approaches each pa-tient, exchanges a couple of words, then injects a needle near the eyes, near the nose, sometimes in the back of the neck, but it ap-pears to be done at random.

He works with astounding speed, injecting about one hun-dred patients per hour, all the while paying seemingly little at-tention to what he is doing. And again, the patients rarely change their facial expressions because they say they feel no pain. Even the children do not cry when the needles are inserted. Dr. Fritz finishes treating more than two hundred patients in about two hours.

It is now the end of the day. Dr Fritz returns to the same chair where he sat eight hours earlier. As he did at the beginning of the day, he covers his eyes with one hand, his head drops down, and Dr. Fritz is gone. Faria is back. He puts on his eyeglasses with the thick lenses. "I am myopic with an astigmatism.

Without these eyeglasses, I am like a blind person. But when I incorporate Dr. Fritz's spirit into myself, he can see everything without glasses, inside and out. I can't explain it. He knows why; I don't know anything about it."

Outside the building, the film crew stops him. Rubens explains that Dr. Fritz's mission is to help people understand a new concept of the spiritual life and to help them live this new life to its fullest measure. "Krishnamurti said, 'There's a great difference between living and experiencing life.' Dr. Fritz wants you to experience your life, so that you can create new guidelines for your life—for why you are living. You can live eighty years and not know how to live those eighty years. There are ten-year-old children who've suffered much more than those eighty-year-olds and already know how to live."

From his office, Neuci Gonclaves, a medical doctor from São Paolo, explains the results of an examination he has conducted. Reading from a medical report, he says, "This is a blood test, CA15.3, that shows breast cancer associated antigens (virus or bacteria) released by tumor cells. The first test shows a level of a hundred and thirty-nine units; of milliliters a normal level is below thirty. Six months after Dr. Fritz's treatments, the patient's new blood test shows a drop to twenty-five units. So this is scientific, material proof that this spiritual treatment is effective."

According to these reports, there have been no errors in the diagnoses or in the treatments Dr. Fritz has given, despite the fact that Rubens is not trained as a doctor and his medical instruments are never sterilized. Rubens explains: "Our margin of

157

error is zero. There have been no proven cases of hospital infection or clinical errors. Nothing. It doesn't exist here. A hospital infection can't happen here because God won't let you get a disease. He only cures. Here the spiritual forces are able to use some sort of energy for sterilization."

Asked why there seems to be no pain when he operates without anesthesia, Rubens-as-Dr. Fritz explains: "I don't use material medicine. I use astral medicine. I'm using my spiritual energy. If you make a map of the brain waves, you'll see that mine and the patient's are very close, the same frequency. That is the theta wave. Then I can promote the liberation of chemical substances in the patient's own body, known as neurotransmitters, specifically endorphins. And faith is a very important factor here. Faith has a mystical esoteric aspect and an energy aspect. When you are able to use this latter aspect, you liberate more endorphins and dopamines. All of these chemical compounds accelerate the higher energy state in your head."

Not only does Dr. Fritz reuse the same syringes over and over all day without sterilizing them, the nurses keep refilling them with the same dark brown liquid, a mixture of alcohol and iodine. "What exactly does this odd concoction do?" he is asked by the interviewer.

"The alcohol in the injection liquid is composed of carbon, hydrogen, and oxygen," Dr. Fritz says. "It's easier to break down these molecules using the raw materials. In reality, the body is not solid. It's an electromagnetic union of particles in constant resonance. When I inject the combination of iodine and alcohol, these substances take on a different configuration inside each person's body, making different substances. I move the magnetic fields. I can use these fields to stop pain and bleeding and to decrease or increase the growth of cells."

He believes that when he injects this liquid into a patient, it goes on a mission to find the diseased cells, then breaks them into individual particles. He can then psychically and energetically reconstruct the remaining healthy particles. And eventually, the once-diseased but now neutralized particles pass naturally, with other waste material, out of the body.

Dr. Fritz claims that he is injecting the energy body, or astral body. "I can't see liver or heart or brain. I just see colors, like the chakras, the same system. The mistake human beings make is that they just focus on the visible body. I see an array of colors that function like the density of water. It's like the phenomenon that happens with the formation of a rainbow. So I am injecting into the astral body, extracting the tumor first from the astral body and second from the material body. In the astral body we don't have pain, bleeding, or infections."

Dr. Fritz offers a self-healing technique for all who are interested. "When I treat patients, I use the energy inside the patient. Everybody has this kind of energy in their cells, inside the mitochondrion (a micro-thread inside the cytoplasm of the cell). The energy I use is closer to the Chinese concept of *chi* energy, or for Indian people, *prana* energy, or what the Japanese call *ki*. But I use this energy very intensively.

159

"I will teach you a simple method to increase your well-being.

First you need to empty your mind. Then imagine and visualize the astral body, which is the same shape as your physical body. Then imagine that astral body filled with golden, shining energy. Next, imagine there is a thick wall on both sides of your body. Then, using the arms and hands of your astral body, try to widen it, and combine this with deep breathing. If you try this, within five minutes you will feel you are getting filled up with invisible, vital energy." He pauses, smiles. "I am here to set you on the road to yourself."

Psychologist Dr. Stanley Krippner of the Saybrook Institute in San Francisco is an outspoken advocate of the work of Rubens Faria. "I think that he's putting on a show that brings out the best in people. Technically, he could do all this without cutting into the skin, without taking on the identity of Dr. Fritz. But that's not the way people's belief systems operate. People like theater, they like spectacle, they like drama, especially people who go to folk healers. Many folk healers around the country tell me, 'I would not have to call on the spirits. I would not have to cut into the body. I would not have to do the rituals, but people expect it, and I must give them what they expect if they are going to be healed.'"

Spiritism came to Brazil in the 1870s, two hundred years after it appeared in the Philippines. Brazil had always had its mystical cults—the *Umbanda* and *Candomble*. As they had in the Philippines, Spanish colonials brought Catholicism. When African slaves arrived, they added their own rituals to the mix.

At the end of the nineteenth century, the works of French

philosopher Alain Kardec and his intellectual doctrine of Spiritism captured the fancy of the Brazilian aristocracy. Kardec's eloquent teachings reflected their own deeply held beliefs in the spiritual realm of existence and paranormal healing performed through mediums.

Again, as in the Philippines, Spiritism drew the fire of the Catholic Church, but eventually the practice found a niche between the Church and the religions of Afro-Brazilians. By the early 1940s, there were more than a thousand Kardecist Spiritist places of worship in Brazil.

Both Brazil and the Phillipines are poor countries that have little or no health care programs. People can barely afford the medical care that is available and their faith is often all they have.

Most of the people who visit these healers seem to accept that not all illness is curable, due to karmic influences, and that a person's illness may be part of their "life lesson." Among those patients who are curable, illness is often seen as a means of raising their belief in God and increasing their level of compassion and love for others.

At the end of the video, Rubens Faria says, "If in every one hundred patients I am able to change the interior of at least one, my work will be accomplished."

# CHAPTER
## SIXTEEN

# JOHN OF GOD,
## THE TAILOR'S SON

A re you going to Brazil?"

"Yes, I plan to. I contacted Rubens Faria, but he's traveling."

"Who's he?"

"He's the medium I want to see."

"What about John of God?"

"Who's he?"

I found myself having the same conversation with just about everyone I talked to in my now well-populated world of healers. I learn that John of God, or Joao de Deus, is a humble man with little or no education, that his father was a tailor and so poor he could barely feed his family. And that Joao has been healing

163

people since the age of sixteen, traveling from village to village, doing his work in exchange for food and shelter. Now, thirty years later, he has his own healing center in central Brazil, where hundreds of thousands of people—rich and poor, movie stars and politicians—from every part of the world have come to be healed by him. He does not charge for his services and only accepts donations that help with the upkeep of the Casa.

I learned more of Joao through Bob Dinga, a Northern Californian whose sight had been restored by John of God. I reached him at his home. It was true, he assured me, and told me the story.

It began in 1986. Bob was at the top of his game as a 38-year-old executive with a multi-million-dollar corporation. Good-looking, house on the beach, luxury car, beautiful wife—life was fine.

Then one morning on his way to the office, Bob lit up his morning cigarette, took a drag, and paused. Tiny pinwheel lights, like Fourth of July sparklers, spun in front of his eyes for just a second, and then they were gone.

Bob forgot about it. But then the tiny lights appeared again, and soon after with greater frequency. Finally, he went to see a doctor. The doctor sent him to an ophthalmologist who sent him to a retinal specialist.

The condition had a name: Serpinous Choroiditis, a rare condition in which the layer behind the retina dies out and scars. Bob's eyesight was steadily deteriorating. For the next twelve years he went from one specialist to another and underwent five laser surgeries. By 1998 he could no longer read, drive a car, or walk unassisted. Bob Dinga was legally blind.

A retinal specialist told him he had better start learning Braille while he still had some vision. Desperate and depressed, Bob sought answers in the alternative medical world—psychics, energy healers, acupuncturists, herbalists, nutritionists. He went to a psychic surgeon in the Philippines, but it was unsuccessful. It seemed he would never get his eyesight back.

Then someone told him about a place in Brazil where people go for miracles. Joao Teixeira da Faria, known as Joao de Deus (John of God) channels *thirty-four* doctors, theologians, and saints. His center, the Casa de San Inacio, is in Abadiania—a tiny, remote village in central Brazil, 103 kilometers from the capital city of Brasilia.

Bob's first day-and-a-half visit at the healing center was too short to make much of a difference in his condition. But subsequent visits of three weeks at a time over the next few months yielded gradual improvement. Each time Bob visited the center, he underwent what he termed "invisible surgeries." After his third visit in 1999, Bob's vision notably improved, and since then his vision has been restored to the point that he can read and drive. He returns to Brazil four times a year now, with his partner Diana, and leads small groups, arranging transportation and lodging. He has made fifteen trips to date.

He explained what invisible surgery was and how it worked, but I confess that what he told me was so incomprehensible, so beyond anything my mind could recognize, that I gave up on a traditional line of questioning. His eye operations, he said, were performed by "entities."

165

I put together a list of people in the U.S. and abroad who have been to see John of God and met with some of them. Some said they had experienced remarkable healings, but *all*—even the most skeptical—said their lives had been forever and dramatically changed.

Alan Cain, a retired builder and painter in his late fifties, was about to have a hip replacement when he happened across an article in a magazine about a psychic surgeon in Brazil. Intrigued, he made some inquiries and decided he had to go.

Alan stayed two weeks. "I saw with my own eyes as Joao, in front of hundreds of people, lifted a woman's blouse, and with what appeared to be a plain kitchen knife, made a small incision in her breast and removed a piece of tissue. When he finished, Joao wiped the blood from the incision on his shirt. The tissue was then sent off to a lab in Brasilia and found to be a cancerous tumor."

Day after day, Alan witnessed events he would never have believed possible: A young French woman with a tumor the size of an orange on her neck was tumor-less after two weeks of treatments; a man from England who had a malignant tumor wrapped around his spine was also cured.

Alan himself had two invisible surgeries for his hip. But he left Brazil disappointed. He had not healed and was still in terrible pain.

After being home for a few days, he noticed that he was climbing the steps in his house without the usual pain. He tried some deep knee bends and squats—exercises he hadn't been able to do for more than two years—and still the pain did not return. The pain was definitely gone.

Curious, Alan went to his doctor and had a repeat CT scan. It showed that the bloodflow to the bone in his hip had not increased. The bone was still essentially dead; he should still be having pain. But he wasn't, and a year-and-a-half later he still isn't having any pain.

Why? Was it the power of his belief at work? Was it that combined with an expectation of a cure based on what he had observed in others? Alan had no explanation. But it happened.

I am told of a doctor who had been hospitalized in Brasilia for a heart condition. Joao rushed to the hospital to attend to him. Five hours after the doctor was declared dead, Joao brought the doctor back to life. I pursue this story and get corroboration from two other people.

I find myself starting to believe things I am not sure I want to believe. Two weeks later, I am on a plane to Brazil.

The trip is long and arduous. From Los Angeles, the flight to São Paulo is nine hours. From São Paulo to Brasilia is another two-hour flight. Then it is an hour-and-a-half drive by taxi, much of it over rough terrain, to Abadiania, where Joao has his Center for Healing.

I'm in the taxi, finally, and the highway climbs through rolling hills dotted with shabby gas stations and dusty villages. Abadiania rests high on a plateau in the state of Goias. I am traveling with Lynn Matis, a psychotherapist from Santa Barbara. A mutual friend had put us in touch. I am grateful; when traveling to another realm, it's reassuring to have a shrink on board.

The houses here are simple, well-kept working-class homes—

167

the sole industry in Abadiania is brick-making. Some are painted bright blue or yellow with red tiled roofs. The colors are vibrant: the iron-rich red earth, cloudless, crystal blue sky. The late-afternoon sun glows neon orange.

The taxi pulls up to our bright blue and white pousada. The driver unloads our bags, but our path is blocked by a column of chickens marching single file along the sidewalk in front of the entrance. "Are they on strike?" I muse aloud.

"They should be," Lynn says. "I hear they're eaten for breakfast, lunch, and dinner."

To keep the population down, I suppose.

Martin comes to greet us. Argentine Martin Mosquera, a thirty-five-year-old former medical student from Buenos Aires, had sustained a severe back injury five years before that would have left him paralyzed but for Joao. Spared a lifetime in a wheelchair, Martin had not only been given a dramatic healing; he had also experienced what he describes as a true state of grace. He stayed on to become one of Joao's translators and eventually to open this pousada where others seeking Joao's help could stay.

He welcomes us with a warm smile and helps with our bags. Inside the gates is a large garden with tables and chairs and a covered veranda for dining. Someone lies in a hammock reading. A boy sits at a table drawing with crayons. A two-year-old chases a spotted dog. Maids chatter in Portuguese. We could be in a sunny resort anywhere in the world.

Martin takes us past a large indoor dining room with six or seven long tables and a self-serve buffet. I stop to look at the photographs tacked onto a bulletin board of the many guests who have stayed here. Pictures of two of the pousada dogs are included with a message: "Chico likes Pedigree Dog Chow, sleeping in the room with you, prefers your bed." The other one, Bono, is called "Stinky" because he likes to roll in cow dung, Martin explains. "He likes to sleep in your room too, but you may want to hose him down first."

My bedroom has two beds. Since there are no shelves, I'll use one bed for my equipment and sleep in the one beneath the window. Next to it is a nightstand made of Formica and molded plastic.

I unpack and have a look around. Outside my bedroom is a small, triangular-shaped garden decorated with bright-colored elves and dancing frogs and polka-dotted mushrooms. Not signs of things to come, I hope.

The pousada is full, an equal mix of Americans and Europeans. There are two families with children. Edwin and Tatiana came from Holland with their eight-year-old son Alexander, the charming, bright boy I had noticed earlier in the garden, who I now see is in a wheelchair. Alexander has Duchaine's Multiple Dystrophy, a serious form of the disease with which he was diagnosed at five. And there is an American, Karen, with her two adopted children, both of whom have brain damage.

The people at the pousada are like characters in a play, each with their own stories and reasons to be in this place at this time. At dinner, I look around the table: A pretty law student at Harvard; a surgical nurse from New Jersey; a male ballet dancer and

169

choreographer with HIV; a wealthy couple from New York; a therapist from London who is thinking of buying a house in Abadiania; a young woman with porcelain skin and large blue eyes who works as a secretary at the World Bank in Belgium; an Asian woman in her thirties with late-stage cancer and her caregiver. Some say they have come for specific healings; others are seeking spiritual growth.

Conversations float back and forth across the dinner table about mysterious and mystical experiences at the Casa, all involving the "entities." I remember hearing this word before from Bob Dinga. The entities are the thirty-four spirit doctors who apparently work through John of God. "Sometimes they start working on you before you get here," someone explains.

"Really?" I ask, struggling to keep an open mind.

One person tells of a "spirit" operation that happened on the airplane on the way down and showed the stitches to prove it. Someone else had an operation while at the waterfall a few miles down the road.

I glance over at the couple from New York. I'm curious to see how hardened New Yorkers are reacting to this, but they are telling their own stories.

I'm exhausted and my back is killing me. Sitting twisted and scrunched in an airplane seat for fifteen hours was not what the doctor ordered. On the way to my room I pass the elves, the rakish frogs, and the polka-dotted mushrooms in the garden again. Yep, and the cow jumped over the moon, I think as I unlock my bedroom door.

There is no bedside lamp. If I want to read, I would have to get out of bed to turn off the overhead light. Instead, I fall asleep with visions of elves and frogs operating on my back.

Sometime during the night I wake to a loud thud. It's me. I'm on the floor. The bed is turned on its side. *Christ, it's an earthquake!* I wait, listening for shouts and sounds of people running, but there is only silence. I get up and turn on the light. The bed frame, made of iron, is upended; the mattress turned lopsided on the floor. I see black marks on the wall where the legs of the bed frame had scraped. *What happened?* I peek out into the hall. All is still.

Terrified, I set the bed back, making sure it's flush against the wall. I put the mattress and bedding back and lie there eyes wide open, listening to the roosters that crow every hour on the hour like church bells, all night long.

Perhaps I dreamt it. In the light of the morning I examine the marks on the wall. The bump on my forehead just above my eyebrow must have come from grazing the corner of the nightstand. Not a dream. I shower and dress and rush out to the dining area. People are lined up at the buffet table. I spot Martin and ask him to please come to my room. I show him the marks on the wall, the bump on my head, and tell him what happened. He nods solemnly. "We'll tell the entity at this morning's session. Get in the *Segundo Vez* line—the second-time line. Don't worry," he adds.

Morning session begins at eight. We have been told to wear white clothing when going to the Casa. We walk along the dusty

171

road in groups of two or three. Locals pass us on bikes or in horse-drawn carts or an occasional truck. Village dogs join the procession, Chico and Bono among them. Shop owners look on from food stalls and roadside shops. Some sit on aluminum chairs on the sidewalk, shaded from the already hot sun.

They must be used to the visitors—the Casa opened over twenty years ago. Still, many of the locals are devout, even fundamentalist, Catholics, and I can't help but wonder how they view this parade of people dressed in white who invade the quiet of their village.

I am walking with Lynn. She notices the bump above my eyebrow and asks about it. I mumble something about walking into a door and change the subject. I am not ready to talk about it.

Alexander and his parents, Edwin and Tatiana, are just ahead. We call out to them and Alexander turns in his wheelchair. "Today is my birthday!" he says in his charming accent. He is smiling happily.

"Well, happy birthday!"

"It is my birthday because today I am going to walk!" Like us, today is his first visit to the Casa. Alexander is convinced Joao will lay his hands on his legs and he will get up out of the wheelchair and walk. Edwin and Tatiana smile bravely, a little apologetically. "Alexander is convinced of this," his mother says. "We try to tell him it may take time." But Alexander raises his arm in victory and hurries them on.

At first, the blue-and-white compound with lines of buses outside looks like a school. The Casa de San Inacio sits at the edge of the village, surrounded by well-tended gardens and covered walkways, overlooking one of the most exquisite valleys I've ever seen. Across the gardens, smaller buildings house a bookshop, dining area, and crystal treatment rooms. The design of the Casa is said to have come to Joao in a vision given to him by his principal entity, Saint Ignatius de Loyola.

The main hall is already crowded with perhaps two hundred people, mostly Brazilians. These are not the very poor seen at Rubens Faria's clinic; these are middle-class people who have come in on buses from around the country. The severity of illnesses and disabilities look the same, though—children with deformed limbs, the blind, the elderly, people in wheelchairs or on crutches. The expressions of hope and expectancy on their faces are the same. They sit squeezed on benches or mill about waiting for the program to begin.

I had noticed on the way in a small room on the right filled with discarded wheelchairs and crutches and in an adjoining room shelf after shelf of eyeglasses, apparently no longer needed.

Volunteers, a few of whom speak English, wear light blue jackets. They show us where to get our tickets, which are free, and where to line up for the "entity room."

My ticket is red and says, "Segundo Vez." Lynn looks at it and tells me I got the wrong one. "We're *Primero Vez,*" she says. I tell her that Martin told me to get this one. I don't know why.

On a raised platform at the end of the hall, a man is speaking into a microphone in Portuguese, explaining the morning's program. On the wall behind him hangs a wooden triangle with folded pieces of paper tucked inside. People wait their turn to stand, pray, and place written requests for blessings inside the triangle. Some lean their foreheads against the center of the triangle and weep. On every wall are paintings of Joao and the entities. I am surprised to see a framed set of pages of Tibetan scriptures on the wall, along with a letter from the Dalai Lama.

A tall, slender man with blue eyes, a beard, and longish light-brown hair takes the microphone. Barefoot, dressed in white, he introduces himself as Ultan. He explains that he first came to the Casa five years ago from his home in Ireland for healing and has never left. He opened an outdoor café down the road from the Casa that serves smoothies and sandwiches. A year later, he married Martin's sister.

In his Irish accent, Ultan translates Joao's message to all who are present today. ". . . This is more than a hospital; this is a spiritual hospital. Here we present more than our physical bodies. We present everything we are; everything we've ever been is here to be healed. The condition of our minds, our emotional life, our hopes for the future, our past lives. Our genetics, relationships with friends and family, our ancestors—all these things make us who we are now. It would be foolish to think these things don't affect each other.

"Maybe it's a physical healing we're looking for, but there may be other aspects of our lives that need healing before a physical healing can happen—other aspects of ourselves we're not aware of that need healing before the healing we're looking for can happen. Healings here are rarely quick, despite what people may hear. There *are* instant healings, but in general healing takes time—we need to make deep changes within ourselves first.

"Try to be open to change in whatever way those changes may come. It may be an opening of our minds, our belief systems, breaking down of our rigidity, forgiveness of old wounds, hurts. It may come as a surprising change in our lives. Rest assured these changes are all for the better, however painful.

"Joao says, 'If you come here with a thimble, that's how much of a blessing you'll get; if you come with a cup, you'll get a cupful of blessing, bring a bowl and you'll get a bowlful. But bring me a swimming pool and you'll get blessings enough to fill the whole pool.'"

We are told that when we pass before Joao-in-entity, we may ask for three healings or answers to questions. In front of me and behind me people desperately ill or crippled wait their turn. Feeling suddenly that I have no right to be in the line, taking up Joao's (or the entity's) time, I step out of the line. Immediately, one of the staff stops me. "I'm just here to learn," I explain.

She smiles and gently leads me back to my place in line. "That's why we're all here." The question foremost on my mind is, Why am I in this "second time" line and does it have something to do with my falling out of bed last night?

The long line files through a room called a *current room*, where thirty or more people are sitting on long benches, their eyes closed in meditation. These people are volunteer mediums who 175 together supposedly generate a powerful healing current. This is one of two current rooms, the other is where Joao-in-entity performs healings.

I notice someone standing to the side filming. I learn later that Joao encourages the video recording of his daily work and welcomes the observation of anyone, especially medical doctors who come to scrutinize the operations. I am told that in forty years there has never been a single case of septicemia in the house. What hospital can make that claim? I am also told that Joao-in-entity operates on more people in one day than many hospitals do in a month. Documentation is limited though. Among the volunteers, only one who devotes two days a week keeps track of records. They are working on improving this system, one of the staff tells me.

When only five or six people remain in front of me, I get my first look at John of God. He is strong-featured, with a heavy frame and longish, black hair, and looks like an ordinary Brazilian workingman: a tailor's son. He sits in a large armchair; flowers and candles are on the table next to him. A woman kneels before him, her head bowed. Joao looks up from the woman and scans the line of people behind her. For just a moment our eyes meet. I have heard that the spirit entities that work through Joao are able to see in one instant a blueprint of each person's life—illness, spiritual evolvement, genetics, ancestral line, past and future.

Joao's eyes are magnified by his glasses. At least that is what I tell myself. And they are a strange, dark blue that shimmer like a child's marble. Or maybe it's the reflection of the candlelight.

When I come face to face with him, it is as if a hundred pairs of eyes are looking at me. Martin is speaking to Joao-in-entity in Portuguese, and Joao is listening, watching me. He nods, asks a question. Martin points to the bruise over my left eyebrow. I want to say, "Forget it, I was probably dreaming; I probably turned over in my sleep really hard and fell onto the floor. I probably just got caught up in all the talk of entities and mysterious visitations." I want to explain that I'm a bit suggestible. I want to say this, but it's too late. Joao has already directed me to go sit on one of the benches in the room and meditate. Martin tells me Joao says the entities will tell me what they want me to know.

Dutifully, I squeeze in between a woman who makes a strange hissing sound as she breathes and an old man who sits motionless. I close my eyes and concentrate on not concentrating. I am not a great meditator; I am very good at daydreaming and watching the colors inside my eyelids. No voices, no messages. But a thought had drifted through my mind that assuming there are such things as entities, perhaps they wanted to make their presence clearly felt to me. If so, they can rest their case.

After a time, I feel movement beside me. The hissing has stopped and the old man is struggling to his feet. The morning session is over. I am surprised to find out I had been sitting there not meditating for almost two hours.

The crowd files out to the covered veranda where volunteers stand at a window ladling out vegetable soup to the hundreds of people lined up, free of charge. Spiritual soup.

I find Lynn. She has come as a "surrogate" for her mother in Colorado who has Alzheimer's. A surrogate presents a photograph to the entity of the person in need of healing but who is unable to make the trip.

"How did it go?" she asks.

"I was sent to go sit in one of the rooms and meditate," I said. "How about you?"

"Joao drew an X on the back of my mother's picture and prescribed some herbs."

A woman across the table says she asked the entity if she would ever find her soul mate. Next to her a man holds his brain-damaged two-year-old in his arms.

We are not here to judge.

I have not seen Alexander and his parents since morning, and I wonder about him. If but one miracle is bestowed on the Casa this day, let it be for Alexander.

The afternoon session begins at two. On the way back to the Casa, I feel a twinge in my back. After my mother's funeral, my back had gotten worse and my doctor insisted I have an MRI. The film showed calcification on my spine, which sometimes pressed on a nerve and caused a fair amount of pain. Sitting twisted and scrunched in an airplane seat for fifteen hours did not help matters. Nor did falling out of bed. My back throbs now as I walk. I have to stop every few minutes and try to stretch it out.

I realize I could present this to Joao and request a healing, but I have a dilemma: I do not like the idea of someone cutting into me with an unsterilized kitchen knife, no matter how spiritually guided that knife may be. Invisible surgeries are more common, I am told, but what if the entity decides I need the real thing?

When I get to the Casa, I ask Martin. He assures me no one gets a visible surgery unless they ask for one, and even then it is up to the entity to decide if it is appropriate.

I walk out onto the promontory and gaze across the valley to the sweeping hills in the distance. I have come to this place not found on any map, where night is day and winter is summer, where butterflies are as big as birds and hummingbirds are the size of robins, where quartz crystals lie in the fields beneath our feet. And last night for the first time ever, I saw the constellation of the Southern Cross. How could I *not* ask to experience a healing?

I get in the afternoon line. When I reach Joao, Martin tells him about my back. "Surgery. Tomorrow morning," Joao says with a wave of his hand. "Eight o'clock."

"But —?"

Joao's attention is already on the person next in line.

The next morning, Thursday, I arrive at the Casa at seven forty-five. My heart pounding, I follow a volunteer staff member to the room adjoining the one where Joao sits. The door is closed. She opens it quietly and directs me past white-sheeted beds lined up against the wall to my seat on one of the padded benches. Among those lying on one of the beds is the young Asian woman from the pousada.

Music plays softly on a tape deck. The staff member tells me

I must sit very still and keep my eyes closed. "Do not cross your arms or legs," she says, "it will block the flow of energy. And do not open your eyes until you are told to."

I remembered what Martin had said about invisible surgeries: Some people feel nothing; some might feel a tingling sensation. The main thing is, stay focused and present. "Do not walk back to the pousada," he said, "take a taxi and go to your room and lie down. You will need to rest for twelve hours. You must treat yourself as if you've had surgery in any hospital."

I take my seat and close my eyes. What happened next wiped all thoughts of placebo or belief or suggestion from my mind. Moments after I sat down, my body went numb. I smelled what I thought must be ether. I could taste it. I recognized the smell and the taste of it from twenty years earlier when I had my appendix removed. I remembered the sensation of being engulfed in a soft blue cloud. I was feeling it again now.

They must be piping anesthesia into the room, I thought. I couldn't help it. I had to peek. I had to see where it was coming from, a hose, a pipe. I glanced at the other people sitting peacefully, eyes closed, hands on their knees. Were they all drugged?

The soft blue cloud closes around me. I am inside it now. I feel nothing.

From a distance, in a language I don't understand, a man's voice intones what sounds like a prayer. I think so because people are joining in. Then I feel a hand on my shoulder. I open my eyes. The woman who had led me in is telling me to get up. Steadying me, she leads me to the door. We file out to the strains of the Beatles' "Strawberry Fields" on the tape deck. "Nothing is real . . ."

Next, I am in a taxi pulling up in front of the pousada. Debby, the surgical nurse, walks me to my room. Eleven hours later I wake up, drink some water, and go back to sleep.

When I next look, it is dawn, six-thirty. Outside my window a rooster and a cow are engaged in a shouting match. A puppy whines. I feel fine. Very well rested.

In the dining room, people are lined up at the breakfast buffet. Eggs, fresh rolls, papaya, pineapple, coffee. I want it all.

"How do you feel?" Debby asks.

"Fine. Great. Thanks for helping me. I was really out of it."

"Of course you were, you had surgery. I know from the O.R. how a person looks after coming out of surgery. What did they operate on?"

"My back, I think."

Debby obviously knows the ropes, not only hospital-wise, but about the Casa, too. She advises me to take it easy, read, hang around. "In a week they'll take out the stitches."

"Who will?"

"The entities. They'll come during the night. Put a glass of water next to your bed on the seventh night. When you wake up, drink it all."

I can't believe I am having this conversation.

"Will it hurt?" I ask.

"No," she says.

"That's good."

This is not a manageable reality, I think.

I lie in the hammock and read Kardec, the French philosopher who introduced Spiritism to Brazil in the 1800s. "... *It is not permitted, at this time, to unveil to you the laws that regulate the gases and fluids by which you are environed; but, before many years have passed, before the space of a human life is accomplished, the explanation of these laws and of these phenomena will be obtained by you; and you will witness the rise of a new variety of mediums . . .*"

Edwin and Alexander come by. I look up from my book as Edwin lifts Alexander out of the wheelchair. Supported by his father, Alexander puts down one foot, then the other.

Excited, I start to get up. Edwin smiles and says, "It's not what you think. We do a little of this every day to exercise the muscles." Alexander is smiling, too. If he was disappointed that he did not get up and walk that first day, he doesn't show it.

"I will walk," Alexander reassures me, as if reading my mind.

His mother, Tatiana, brings out balloons. Today is both Edwin's and Martin's birthday and tonight there will be a party.

In most countries it is customary to send a birthday card; in Brazil they send a birthday *car*. Large, brightly decorated with flashing red lights, music blaring the fast beat of Brazilian pop, the car comes rolling through the gates right into the garden. Everyone dances. Several small children make a line and do what looks like a perfectly choreographed dance.

A shout goes up. A beautiful horse is being led through the garden gates, a gift to Martin from his family. Martin grabs his two-year-old son and climbs up onto the horse's back. In the middle of all this, a man with longish black hair and glasses has come in. He hugs Martin. Then he sits on one of the lawn chairs and watches the dancing. It is Joao.

Martin introduces me. He tells him I am writing a book on healing. Joao smiles and nods. "What would you like to know?" he asks.

"I guess what I would most like to know is, what must it be like to be Joao?"

His answer, translated by Martin, is in Joao's own words. "I never healed anybody; who heals is God. I am only an instrument with many faults, a very small instrument. I received this mission when I was nine years old and started when I was sixteen. I am a person who did not have the opportunity of an education. But I have this mission that has gone on for more than forty years. I will continue on until the end of my forces.

"I know all the states from Brazil, all the important capital cities, but here in this small city of Abadiania I am here for more than twenty-three years. When people ask, 'Are you Joao the tailor, Joao the construction worker, Joao the son of Jose Nunes da Faria?' I say 'Yes, I'm that Joao.'

"What makes my mission beautiful is when somebody comes and tells me that they received a cure or a relief. I know that it all comes from the power of God. My mission is not to create any kind of religion or cult; the only thing that I want is for the entire world to believe in the Creator of the universe. This energy comes from Him who heals. Our mission in our lifetime is 183 to respect and love that energy, God's energy."

Joao seems a little surprised by all the fuss made over him. As an "unconscious medium," he has no memory of the healings and the operations that are done through him. When he is told of some miracle that occurred while he was "incorporated," he is glad.

He smiles now, enjoying the music and watching the children dance. Fernanda, Martin's wife, and his cousins who have come from Argentina cook hot dogs and hamburgers over an open fire. Joao gratefully accepts a hot dog. Joao clearly loves Martin, and Martin speaks about Joao with unrestrained trust and belief in what he does and who the man is.

The story goes that Joao's gift came to him at the age of sixteen in a vision. He had been wandering jobless and hungry when he heard a woman call his name. Out of the shadows a fair-haired woman appeared and told him, "Go to the Redemptor Spiritual Center, they are waiting for you there." When he got there, an elderly priest greeted him, and asked to come inside.

Joao did not remember the next few hours. He thought he had fainted from hunger. When he came to, he was told that he had performed a miraculous operation on a woman and healed her of an incurable disease.

As Joao tells it, when he went outside, he found a crowd of people all waiting to be healed. Later, he learned that the woman who had come to him in a vision and directed him to the church was Saint Rita of Cassia, the patron saint of Brazil.

For the next eight years, Joao traveled from town to town, healing the sick in exchange for food and shelter. Word of his healings spread and eventually reached the authorities. Everywhere Joao went police found him, arrested him, threw him into prison, and beat him. Finally, Joao took a job with the military in Brasilia as a civilian tailor where, under the army's protection, he could continue healing. Nine years later, Joao had saved enough money to buy a small farm. The farm turned out to be rich in minerals and gems, and in 1978 Joao was able to establish the center in Abadiania.

The authorities continue to pursue him. Police regularly appear with warrants for his arrest. In 1995 Joao's lawyers appeared before a Supreme Court Judge who had received an operation from Joao-in-entity and who pointed out that ". . . acts performed by incorporated entities were not crimes."

Another Supreme Court judge in São Paulo stated, "In the existence of quackery the presence of fraud is presupposed, which cannot happen to the mediumized individual. This last, in a state of trance, finds himself unconscious and therefore may not be held responsible for actions undertaken in his absence by the spirits incorporated by him."

On one of my last days in Abadiania, I saw three armed policemen enter the hall and thought I was about to witness one of these arrests. Instead, the three, one a woman, got into the line with everyone else. They were there for a healing.

In the two weeks I had been there, I had seen a woman add her eyeglasses to the discarded eyeglass collection and a man leave his wheelchair behind in the room for discarded wheelchairs and crutches.

185

Edwin, Alexander's father, left his job in Holland and rented a house across the street from Martin's. Alexander continues to make progress, slowly gaining strength in his muscles. They will stay in Abadiania for several more months.

The morning of my last day, I go to the Casa to say good-bye and to take flowers to Joao. I see the staff member who had helped me during my surgery and we stop to talk. She had heard about the incident in my room my first night. Whether she had discussed it with Joao or not, the reason to her was clear: I had come not only as a journalist but for my own healing as well. And for both reasons, the entities wanted to make their presence known to me.

Rather rudely, I thought, and said as much.

"For some, subtle messages are likely to be reasoned away."

Point well taken.

My back is much better and I promise myself one day I will have another MRI. For the moment though, I am able to sit at my desk without pain. I am grateful for the healing, whether the work of elves or entities.

# EPILOGUE

Brazil is fading fast; I am back in the modern realm. Streets are clogged with cars instead of chickens. Jets streak across a pale sky, and birds and butterflies have shrunk to their normal size.

I pick up the morning newspaper: the world in black and white. It needs healing. Not surgeries, unless they're invisible, not chemicals, and certainly no more radiation. It needs armies of entities and commanders like Vianna and Howard. It needs Warren to teach everyone to sing. If Dr. Ruth were Prime Minister of the universe, no one would be allowed to store tension. Gerry and his Mob could give folks on the other side of the pond a good Bundjalung Tickle.

One newspaper article in particular catches my eye, a study by the Institute of Medicine reported in the *New York Times*. According to that study, medical mistakes kill up to 98,000 hospitalized patients each year. The report included only those incidents occurring in hospitals, not incidents occurring outside hospital care.

The results energy healers or psychic surgeons achieve cannot be quantified; they have no means or methods of keeping track of the thousands of people who come seeking their help each year. Those who have been healed might write a testimonial as a form of thanks; those who have not been healed are generally never heard from again.

Healers don't usually kill anyone. Except maybe with false hope, as in the case of the actor who refused medical treatment and put himself in the hands of the Chinese healer I met in Denver. Some said the actor died of his own gullibility.

Who are the people who turn to healers? The ones I met and interviewed were those who had broken faith with the doctors who had given up on them. Their diseases were too far advanced, they were told, or there was no known cure for their particular disease. Or, in the case of Amy, told she must resign herself to spending the rest of her life as a "talking head" encased in a block of ice.

Sometimes what they had was nameless. Nothing medically wrong. Stress, perhaps. (Here, take one of these every day with breakfast.) Or an inchoate emptiness, an unnamed fear, lack of purpose, a feeling of un-connectedness. Fatigue? Can't sleep? Can't get going in the morning? Try one of these.

So they turned to healers for hope. I am reminded of the principle of the placebo effect: Hope plus belief equals expectation, which in many cases can trigger healing—sometimes called a spontaneous remission, sometimes called a miracle. Some report a feeling of ecstasy, a religious experience. Like falling in love.

Some, the spiritually hungry, look to healers to help them find a purpose, a reason.

It has been said that a good healer, a truly inspired healer, has the ability to reconnect us with our own life force, which hungers for wholeness in the same way a houseplant turns its face toward the sun. Something modern science, with all its astounding medical breakthroughs, cannot do. Curing versus healing.

"Healing is just one of God's parlor tricks," Howard Wills once said, "to prove the existence of the Divine."

I often asked, what about the ones who are not healed—even by the most gifted healers? Gerry Bostock says, "Their illness serves them in some way, gets them the attention they need." Peter Maxwel says, "For some I just don't have the key to unlock whatever it is that keeps them sick."

And then there is always the Karma Defense.

Looking back, I realize that all of the healers I met have their own personal version of God, each with a different face. Sandra    189

Ingerman's god, the one she glimpsed during her two near-death experiences, loves unconditionally, without prejudice, sinners and saints alike. Howard Wills' god demands prayers, eight twice a day, while the god Vianna speaks to responds to direct commands. Virginia's high-pitched call must pierce the heavens, while Warren's god heals with the help of equipment and Warren's heart, which is the size of an elephant's. Gerry's Mob runs his show, and Katie's god showers her with flakes of gold.

But to watch John of God with his army of entities is to have one's whole system of belief forever changed.

I have often been asked, given what I have seen as a traveler between realms, if I had it to over again when I was diagnosed with a show-stopping illness in 1991, or if I had a recurrence now, what I would do. My answer is—everything. First, I would go to the white-coated wizards and take whatever help they had to offer. Then I would go to the doctors of soul and spirit and get healed.